MULTIPLE PERSONALITY
An excercise in deception

MULTIPLE PERSONALITY
An excercise in deception

Ray Aldridge-Morris

Principal Lecturer in Psychopathology
Middlesex Polytechnic School of Psychology

Sessional Chartered Clinical Psychologist
Princess Alexandra Hospital, Harlow

LEA LAWRENCE ERLBAUM ASSOCIATES, PUBLISHERS LEA
Hove and London (UK)   Hillsdale (USA)

Copyright © 1989 by Lawrence Erlbaum Associates Ltd.
All rights reserved. No part of this book may be reproduced in any
form, by photostat, microform, retrieval system, or any other
means without the prior written permission of the publisher.

Lawrence Erlbaum Associates Ltd., Publishers
27 Palmeira Mansions
Church Road
Hove
East Sussex, BN3 2FA
U.K.

British Library Cataloguing in Publication Data

Aldridge-Morris, Ray
Multiple personality. 1. Multiple personality
I. Title
616.85'236

ISBN 0-86377-128-9

Printed and bound by BPCC Wheatons, Exeter

DEDICATION

To Kathryn, Charlotte and Karen

Contents

Acknowledgements

I welcome this opportunity to express my thanks to all those without whose support this monograph would not have been possible. It was written during a sabbatical year awarded by Middlesex Polytechnic and I am deeply grateful to Professor David Marks not only for his constant encouragement and insightful criticism but also for his valued friendship.

Thanks are also due to Professor Emeritus Peter McKellar, Dr Tom Fahy and two anonymous previewers for their exhaustive critical appraisals of my first draft. Their comments led to many revisions although responsibility for the final version must remain mine.

I have also learned much from discussions with John Davis, John Ives, Noel Lee, Hugh Tollington, David Vinney and Grenville Wall. I am especially indebted to the library staff of Enfield College, in particular, Cathy McGowan, for their invaluable help in my literature search and the collection of more than 350 books and articles.

All this academic support notwithstanding, I could never have completed this project without the love and support of my family. Karen was obliged to share the first year of our marriage with a frequently absent and distracted husband and Kelly, Nicola and Antman had to share their new stepfather with his Amstrad. Mercifully, the marriage seems to have survived.

Far from least, I am forever grateful to my daughters, Kathryn and Charlotte, and my parents, Brenda and Tom, for their unstinting interest and encouragement. I hope they are as proud of me as I am of them.

CHAPTER 1

Splitting Images

In 1957 Thigpen and Cleckley published a book which was to become a landmark in the psychological literature, *The Three Faces of Eve*. This book, and shortly afterwards the film of the same title, brought to the attention of a still increasing lay audience the phenomenon of multiple personality. Based on their original journal article (Thigpen and Cleckley, 1954), the book tells of a patient, dubbed Eve White, from Augusta, Georgia. She was in therapy because of "severe and blinding headaches (and) blackouts" (Thigpen and Cleckley, 1954). After a number of interviews she complained of amnesia for a recent trip but this responded promptly to hypnosis. Some days later an unfinished letter arrived at their office which, although unsigned, was clearly from Eve White. However, it seemed as if someone else had added a few inconsequential lines at the bottom. On her next visit Eve denied sending the letter although she remembered having begun it. As the interview progressed her normal composure slowly disappeared. She became agitated and at one point volunteered she sometimes heard an imaginary voice. Then, Thigpen and Cleckley write "after a tense moment of silence, her hands dropped. There was a quick reckless smile and, in a bright voice that sparkled, she said, 'Hi there, Doc!'." The demure and introverted young woman seemed to have another personality, bright and bouncy, feckless and flirtatious, whose identity was announced as Eve Black.

Thigpen and Cleckley were conspicuously overwhelmed with the separateness of this second personality to the point where scientific precision and objectivity in reporting were somewhat sacrificed. For example, they write that "A thousand minute alterations of manner, gesture, expression, posture, of nuances in reflex or instinctive reaction, of glance, of eyebrow tilting and eye movement, all argued that this could only be another woman. It is not possible to say just what all these differences were .... We are not able to tell adequately what so profoundly distinguishes from Eve White the carefree girl who took her place in this vivid mutation." Robert Louis Stevenson

1

had given the world of fiction Dr Jekyll and Mr Hyde and now Thigpen and Cleckley had presented the world of science with Eve White and Eve Black.

Over the ensuing fourteen months, and 100 hours of interviews, a further personality, Jane, was to emerge. It was later revealed (Lancaster, 1958) that a further nineteen personalities were to manifest themselves after Eve had been discharged. We learn that Eve eventually integrated these twenty two personalities and, under her true identity, Chris Sizemore, became a writer, artist and lecturer (Sizemore and Pitillo, 1977).

Eve was far from the first documented case of multiple personality. Indeed, she had a fair number of historical antecedents dating back more than three centuries. Bliss (1980) reports that the philosopher and physician, Theophrastes Paracelsus (1646), "noted a case in which the personality pilfered her own money, while the subject remembered nothing about it." We know nothing more about this early case but some of the ancestral giants of psychology and psychiatry have written about multiple personality patients from personal experience (James, 1890; Binet, 1896; Prince, 1906; McDougall, 1926).

One case study since Eve has become equally famous, appearing in both book (Schreiber, 1973) and film format, the eponymous "Sybil". Like Eve, she had a multiplicity of personalities, sixteen in all; and, like Eve, she is now reported as integrated, and a lecturer.

More recently, Confer and Ables (1983) have produced a third book-length account of a case of multiple personality, Rene, who allegedly had five alternate personalities.

Taylor and Martin (1944) reviewed the literature more than 40 years ago to reveal 76 cases but they caution that the absence of a precise definition of multiple personality meant that "perhaps no two students in combing the literature would draw up identical lists of cases." Their caution is well advised because producing a rigorous definition of multiple personality presents particular difficulties. Not only are we hampered by the lack of a universally acceptable definition of "personality" but also the very notion of "multiple personality" seems to strike at the core of a fundamental belief about the nature of human beings, namely, that we are internally consistent. Of course, this does not deny the commonplace observation that people can behave unpredictably even to the point of apparent contradiction. However, appearances can deceive and we are likely to dismiss behavioral inconsistency as superficial, as belying a basic unity of the personality. We are very adept at dealing with contrary evidence in order to preserve fundamental beliefs. Festinger's theory of "cognitive dissonance" and Anna Freud's "ego-defense mechanisms" are two notable examples of psychology's attempt to explore this human propensity. We should not be surprised at our acquisition of such coping strategies since they are essential to the maintenance of our psychic equilibrium. A world where all seemed totally random would be as unbearable as one where total predictability reigned. We have a basic human need to make sense of what William James so memorably dubbed the "booming, buzzing confusion" of life and Sir Frederick Bartlett has similarly laid stress on our constant "efforts after meaning". Our physical survival depends on our learning strategies to ward off aggression, combat disease, protect our young and fill our bellies. Our mental stability, in the end, our sanity, requires strategies to cope with the unpredicted and the dissonant. Such strategies, whilst preserving "peace of mind" may none the less involve us in self-deception and the distortion of reality. In our examination of multiple personality we must be as much on our guard against oversimplification, in the service of making the unfamiliar familiar, as we must against overelaboration because of its seductive novelty.

There are those, however, who would question whether my use of the word "novelty" is any longer appropriate since Eve, Sybil and Rene, and the 76 cases collated by Taylor and Martin would seem to be only the tip of an iceberg. Greaves (1980) notes that a further fourteen cases were recorded in the 25 years following Taylor and Martin's review, six of them diagnosed and treated by Dr Cornelia Wilbur, Sybil's psychotherapist. After what might be regarded as a relative slump in the incidence of multiple personality, Greaves goes on to cite at least 50 cases reported during the 70s. One begins to see why Boor (1982) chose to entitle his paper "The Multiple Personality Epidemic."

The following year, Boor and Coons (1983) produced a valuable, classified bibliography comprising 350 references pertaining to multiple personality. Within 2 years this was subjected to a major revision (Damgaard et al., 1985). No less than four journals have published special issues exclusively devoted to multiple personality (*American Journal of Clinical Hypnosis*, 1983; *Psychiatric Annals*, January, 1984; *Psychiatric Clinics of North America*, March, 1984; *International Journal of Clinical and Experimental Hypnosis*, April, 1984). Then, in 1985 a series of 309 multiple personality patients was presented by as many therapists (Schultz et al., 1985). As the number of reported cases mount, and the literature grows, it is none the less puzzling that personal experience of these patients seems to be confined to relatively few clinician/investigators whose names will constantly recur throughout this book.

Kluft (1986), for example, reports that at least ten individuals or groups report seeing series of ten such patients, and Kluft himself has seen a staggering 171 cases, 117 of whom he has treated personally (Coons, 1986).

One could readily say more about recent, pertinent book publications (e.g. Hilgard, 1977; McKellar, 1979; and Bliss, 1986), and about special courses and a society launched to study this phenomenon. There is even a newsletter called "Speaking for Our Selves" which its editorial staff describe as "by, for, and about people with multiple personalities", first issued in October, 1985. However, it must already be abundantly apparent that in the United States, at least, multiple personality is no longer regarded merely as an item of exotica pathologica, still less as mere artefact or "myth".

So, what exactly is the nature of this bizarre and striking syndrome? How may it be defined and classified, and are there sub-classifications? What do we know about its incidence and prevalence? What is known about its aetiology and prognosis? For what signs and symptoms should the diagnostician be alert? What problems of differential diagnosis are posed? Given the steady increase in the number of cases reported by highly qualified and experienced clinicians, how tenable is a sceptical view of this putative disorder? These are the obvious questions provoked by multiple personality to be considered later. Other, more contentious issues will also receive attention.

It will be argued that there is considerable room for scepticism and that, even if multiple personality passes muster as a discrete psychiatric syndrome, it has been grossly overdiagnosed. It will also be suggested that multiple personality is heavily dependent upon cultural influences for both its emergence and its diagnosis.

However, I shall first introduce briefly some of the more famous personalities themselves without critical comment or analysis. (Reference will be made to many other alleged multiple personalities as the book progresses.) At this stage, readers may care to look for common features in the histories and to formulate their own initial hypotheses. The cases chosen are those that have been most fully documented and, relatedly, have acted as landmarks in the history of multiple personality; Eve, Sybil and Rene, together with the earliest figure to receive such thorough description, Miss Beauchamp (Prince, 1906). Although female cases predominate, I also present two men, Billy Milligan and Kenneth Bianchi. Both are convicted offenders who entered pleas of diminished responsibility by dint of being multiple personalities but, as we shall see, only Milligan was successful.

Christine Beauchamp (Prince, 1906)

The first book-length account of multiple personality was "Dissociation of a Personality" (Prince, 1906) and counts as a classic in the literature. It recounts the case of a 23 year old, Radcliffe College, student whose real name was Clara Fowler. In 1898, she came to see Morton Prince, an eminent Boston professor of "nervous diseases", with a history of neurasthenic ailments. She complained of headaches and sleeplessness, lassitude and weight loss, bodily pains and apathy. Her premorbid personality was described as diligent, moralistic and secretive as well as timid and introverted. A pleasant, non-smoking and religious young woman, she was proficient in short-hand, a fluent French-speaker and an avid reader. She also exhibited strong intrapunitive tendencies, indulging in fasts and vigils when pricked by conscience. She had an unhappy childhood which included losing her mother when she was 13, and a succession of traumas which resulted in once running away from home.

Faced with this intelligent and anxious patient, Prince, along with automatic writing and crystal-gazing, chose to employ hypnosis and found her a good subject. However, under hypnosis she presented only her original self, albeit a little less inhibited. None the less, after some weeks, his hypnotherapy seemed to reveal a new, formerly covert personality, who called herself "Sally". Sally seemed to be all that Christine (Prince's pseudonym for Clara) was not. She denied any knowledge of short-hand or French, was extraverted and seductive, smoked and played practical jokes. Christine denied all knowledge of Sally's existence but Sally was aware of Christine to the extent that she was the frequent target of Sally's mischievous humour. For example, Sally would strip naked and strike up a model's pose in her room, only then to "leave", when a very embarrassed Christine would "arrive". Sally would make dates with boyfriends whom

Christine no longer wished to see, and unpick knitting which Christine had spent the night completing. Once she sent Christine, who was arachnophobic, a box of spiders through the post. However, Sally could also be more than helpful. Prince reports that she once intervened to prevent Christine's suicide by switching off the gas. It seems that, mischievous though she was, Sally had a certain appeal, and Prince makes no secret of his ambivalent feelings towards her.

Brief though this résumé must be, it must include reference to a further personality that was to emerge during hypnotherapy. This was a regressive, child-like and ill-tempered personality (Prince dubbed it "the Devil" in contrast to Christine's "Saint" and Sally's "the Woman"). Sally was equally contemptuous of this personality who at one stage was christened "the Idiot", and it, too, was the frequent victim of her pranks, as much the victim of Sally's contempt for its stupidity as was Christine for her primness. Christine was amnesic for this personality as she was for Sally.

Although Clara Fowler's alter egos first appeared during hypnosis it seems they eventually "popped out" spontaneously, alternating as to who had executive control, and occasionally creating a comedy of errors.

Throughout Prince's account, Sally emerges as the dominant force and Prince saw one of his therapeutic tactics as the "squeezing out" of this personality although she played a frequent role as "observer" and therapist's aide, providing information about episodes for which Christine was amnesic. The "cure" of Clara Fowler resided in the reconciliation of her original personality and the final, regressive, personality which emerged. Miss Fowler was later to marry an assistant of Prince.

During therapy Prince was active in christening the emergent personalities and he corresponded with them separately. He also made no secret of his preference for Sally who became pre-eminent. The question is raised, therefore, of an iatrogenic component in Miss Fowler's presentation.

Eve (Thigpen and Cleckley, 1954, 1957; Sizemore and Pittillo, 1977)

Despite the striking aspects of this case history, recorded, as it was, by a noted professor, it seems to have attracted little scientific attention until "Eve" arrived on the professional scene some 50 years later. Eve's is a considerably more complex, and more fully documented case. Aged 25, and a telephonist with a modest educational background ("she quit high-school 2 months before graduating"), Eve presented with a history of severe headaches, black-outs and amnesic episodes. She came from a loving, even overprotective family environment, and was born 2 months prematurely to poor South Carolina tenant farmers. Her family was very close, her aunt and uncle being the sister and brother of her parents. When their own child, Eve's cousin, died in early infancy they formed an especially close bond of love with their niece.

Of doubtless significance in her childhood, she witnessed a drowned corpse in a nearby ditch, and was told by her mother, Zueline, that a monster was responsible; a monster that would harm Eve were she to trespass near the water herself. In her autobiography Christine Sizemore (Eve) reports that, at the time of the discovery of the corpse, she thought she saw a red-haired girl standing on the bridge. Although now a brunette, Eve had been born with red hair and nick-named "Carrot Top" as a child. She reports that she saw the red-haired stranger later when her mother cut herself badly on a broken jar and Eve thought she was going to die. If these two events were not enough, Eve was later to see the victim of a saw-mill accident, a man severed into three segments.

Eve is described as a plain little girl and jealous of other children, including twin sisters born when she was 6 years old. However, she came to be very close not only to her twin sisters but also to her cousin, Elen, who was 3 years her junior. Throughout her childhood she was frequently accused of malicious acts against her peers and animals but always attributed responsibility to another, "ugly"girl, and became known as a liar.

She grew into an attractive young woman but entered unknowingly into a bigamous marriage with a racing driver. He was a brutal, hard-drinking sadist, insisting on anal intercourse and she eventually left him and returned to her parents. Later she met a soldier, Ralph White, but he was a boring and mechanical lover who showed little tenderness or interest in his wife. When Eve gave birth to a daughter they argued as to whether she should be brought up in Ralph's Catholic faith. At this time she reported hearing voices which expressed her hostility towards her boring husband, and her behaviour began to give him increasing cause for concern. For example, her voices urged her to "knock his block off!" and, as he stood shaving in front of the bathroom mirror, to "pull that rug from under him." Compliance with her voices led her once to pull the tablecloth from under a meal he was eating, spilling food all over Ralph. On other occasions she was incontinent during rows with him. By now the marriage was doomed and she again returned to her parents' home, and it was from there she was referred to Dr Corbett Thigpen.

Thigpen also employed hypnosis and found he could "call out" Eve Black quite readily after she had made her initial appearance as described in the opening of this chapter. What struck him was the sharp contrast between the demure and conservative Eve White, and the provocative, even coarse Eve Black. (In fact, the names used were Chris White and Chris Costner, her maiden name.) Eve Black always insisted on being referred to as "Miss" and was scornful of Eve White, a wife and mother. She took great pleasure in Eve White's embarrassment at finding in her wardrobe loud dresses which had been bought while Eve Black had been "out" on a shopping expedition. However, she is also reported as having foiled a suicide bid by Eve White, when she caused her to drop the razor she was holding. Thigpen reports that Eve Black said, "I think she meant business, Doc."

Later, a third personality, Jane, emerged and had the appearance of a more calm and mature personality. Chris Sizemore reveals that she based Jane's name on "Jane Eyre". It became Thigpen's goal to fade out the two Eves to allow Jane to take control and, by now, he was treating this fascinating patient free of charge. In time he seemed to have achieved this goal, and Jane had met Don Sizemore, who had asked her to marry him. Chris Sizemore writes that when she told Thigpen about her marriage plans Thigpen replied, "I have a very warm feeling for you, Jane, ... I love you Jane." (This is a little reminiscent of Prince's declared fondness for Sally.) At this Jane replied "Oh, I'm so sorry, Dr Thigpen. I'm so sorry." Jane was discharged and married soon after and Thigpen was not to know that 19 more personalities were to yet to appear. For example, there was one obsessed with collecting bells, another who was blind, a third who was fascinated by turtles, another by things purple, and yet another who loved strawberries. Chris Sizemore spent 20 more years seeing psychiatrists and producing personalities and the interested reader can find the full account in her book, written with her cousin Elen Pittillo.

Sybil (Schreiber, 1973)

Sybil Dorsett (a pseudonym) was a 22-year-old postgraduate when she sought help from Dr Cornelia Wilbur in New York. A distinctive feature is that the only, albeit very full, record of this case is a book by Schreiber, a professor of English and Speech and a former psychiatry editor of a publication called "Science Digest". Surprisingly, Dr Wilbur has not gone into print, herself, concerning this dramatic case although she introduced Schreiber to the patient and vouched for the accuracy of the final version of Schreiber's account.

Sybil had a history of amnesic episodes, bad headaches and hysterical blindness. Her childhood was nothing short of horrendous. Her father was a relatively affluent building contractor and her mother a talented pianist, but whilst her father was at work, Sybil was subjected to physical and sexual abuse of an extraordinary nature. She would be tied to the legs of the piano while her mother played and strung up by light flex, legs apart, when her mother would fill her vagina with cold water. Her ostensibly prudish parents would also make love in full view of their daughter who shared their bedroom until she was 9 years old.

Schreiber reports that Sybil had an imaginary playmate, Vicky, who lived a sophisticated life in Paris. It seems that even in childhood yet another personality emerged, this time "unbidden", namely "Peggy Lou". Peggy Lou was a "stand-up-and-fight" character whose existence seemed to be a reaction to her mother's aggression and it was she who first presented herself as an alter-ego to Dr Wilbur. Suddenly, one day in analysis, Sybil began talking in a childish and ungrammatical voice and Vicky was not far behind in revealing her "presence".

Wilbur used both hypnosis and drug abreaction during her psychoanalytically based therapy. As time went on a further 13 personalities were to present themselves including Peggy Ann who resembled Peggy Lou but without the anger; Mary Lucinda who was homeloving and motherly; Ruthie, who was a baby; Marcia who was a writer and artist; Mike and Sid who were carpenters; and Marjorie who was a serene and vivacious "tease". "Vanessa" alone could play the piano. Sybil reported different body images for her various personae so that, for example, Mary had long, brown hair, and Marjorie was a willowy brunette. Mike was brown eyed and olive skinned whereas Sid was fair skinned with blue eyes.

In some cases the source of the personalities was clear. For example, one could recognise Sybil's grandmother in Mary, and Sybil's father in the carpenters.

There was a complex amnesic relationship between the personalities with Sybil being primarily unaware of her different selves but, generally, they all got on well with each other. It seems that Vicky was the most "co-conscious" personality, being in touch with most of what was going on in the other personalities. Wilbur actively used her as "co-therapist" since Vicky distanced herself from what she saw as the neurotic Sybil, a personality she felt she could assist from afar.

Sybil spent 11 years in therapy with Wilbur who resolved her patient's multiplicity by fusing all personalities into one.

Rene (Confer and Ables, 1983)

Rene is a relatively recent case who was seen in 1978 aged 27 with a history of two overdoses. She complained of memory lapses, suicidal thoughts, derealisation and said that, when a teenager, she had heard voices ("a bunch of people talking low"). She had suffered horribly at the hands of her parents. Her alcoholic father had raped her when she was 11, and her mother had pressed her to cunnilingus. As a child Rene was locked in a wardrobe, beaten and burned with a cigarette.

Rene's mother was promiscuous and it was during Rene's account of her mother's extramarital relations that she began having breathing difficulties and she said she felt as if the seat of a stool was pressing against her chest. At this point, Confer and Ables report that "Jeane", an alternate personality appeared. Jeane was a spunky 19 year old, assertive, and tom-boyish. Four other personalities eventually appeared: Stella was 18, sultry and seductive but unable to give love; Sissy Gail was a tearful and abused 4 year old who adopted a fetal crouch; Bobby was a 20 year old male friend of Rene's two brothers and bent on murderous revenge; Mary was the last personality to emerge and is described as a "holy roller".

Confer and Ables conducted a number of personality assessments using the MMPI and the results are reported in Chapter 5. Distinctively, these authors report "successful merging of all alternates" after little more than 3 months therapy which involved not only hypnosis but also enlisted the aid of members of Rene's family.

Billy Milligan (Keyes, 1981)

Billy Milligan was convicted of rape at the age of 23. His natural father committed suicide when Billy was three and his mother, who had two other children, later married for the first time but this lasted only 2 years. She married again, this time to a religious fanatic who beat Billy mercilessly and subjected him to anal intercourse. As an adolescent Billy evidenced trances and minor fugues as well as aphonia. He joined the navy at 17 but was discharged as unsuitable after only a month. Soon after he served a year in prison for rape and later committed further robberies and assaults, abusing drugs along the way, until his notable court appearance in Columbus, Ohio, following a series of rapes in 1977.

It transpired that Billy had ten personalities, one of whom, "Arthur", aged 22, planned the rapes. Only Arthur was aware of all the other personalities. Another personality described as an aggressive "keeper of hate", Ragan, initiated the assaults but the actual rapist was a lesbian personality, aged 19, named Adalena. Other personalities to emerge were Allen, aged 18, an artist and drummer; Tommy, aged 16, Danny, aged 14, and Christopher, aged 13, who were quiet and timid; David, aged 9, who was depressive and autistic; and Christine, aged 3, who craved affection and liked painting.

Billy was found not guilty on grounds of insanity and was confined to a maximum security prison hospital where he established something of a reputation as a gifted artist. He has since been discharged to outpatient status.

It only remains to make a preliminary reference to Kenneth Bianchi, like Milligan, a convicted rapist. However, his tale takes on even more serious proportions in that he was also a multiple murderer. Bianchi's case remains controversial today and several distinguished psychopathologists are involved. Owing to the degree of scholarly attention accorded to this case, and the provocatively divided opinion as to diagnosis, the following chapter is devoted to its presentation.

Hopefully, the reader will now have at least a descriptive acquaintance with a handful of some of the more notable cases of multiple personality. There will be further reference to these cases, along with many others as the book progresses but it seems opportune to say something now about the attempts at formal definition and classification.

Taylor and Martin (1944) defined multiple personality as "one human being demonstrating two or more personalities with identifiable, distinctive and consistently ongoing characteristics, each of which has a relatively separate memory of its life history. ... There must also be a demonstration of the transfer of executive control of the body from one personality to the other (switching). However, the total individual is never out of touch with reality. The host personality (the one who has executive control of the body the greatest percentage of the time during a given time) often experiences periods of amnesia, time loss or black-outs. Other personalities may not experience this."

The omission of amnesia as a defining characteristic is striking in the current, third edition of the American Psychiatric Association's Diagnostic and Statistical Manual of Mental Disorders (DSM III, 1980). Here, for the first time, multiple personality enjoys the status of a discrete, diagnostic entity under the dissociative disorders. In the previous edition, DSM II (1963), there was no description of multiple personality which was subsumed under hysterical neurosis, dissociative type.

In DSM III (p. 257) it is defined as the "Existence within an individual of two or more distinct personalities, each of which is dominant at a particular time. The personality dominant at any particular time determines the individual's behavior. Each individual personality is complex and integrated with its own unique behavior patterns and social relationships."

Coons (1984), however, immediately follows his quotation of DSM III's criteria with the stricture, "An absolute essential criterion for the diagnosis of multiple personality is the presence of amnesia. Usually the original personality is amnesic for the other secondary personalities."

Clearly, the definition of multiple personality is not without controversy. How essential is amnesia to the diagnosis, and note how DSM III insists that the alternate personalities be complex, functional unities? If the criteria of complexity and integration is adhered to, is it possible to conceive of an individual having a dozen or more personalities? Could one distinguish them from each other? Coons (1980) answers that "Up to 50 personalities have been reported in one person but these individuals contain many short-lived personalities or incompletely formed personality fragments." "Reported" or not, this sounds as if they were not personalities in the sense intended by DSM III.

Coons (1984), once again does not seem unduly restricted by DSM III. As well as insisting on the addition of amnesia to its criteria he goes on to state that "It is a mistake to consider each personality totally separate, whole or autonomous. The other personalities might best be described as personality states, other selves, or personality fragments." The waters of definition are becoming a little muddied. Matters are not helped by the absence of a consensus amongst psychologists as to what is meant by that ubiquitous term "personality". None the less, one's conceptual taste-buds will begin to detect the flavour of this putative syndrome, and the absence of precise definitions has never hampered psychopathologists from delineating signs and symptoms for which the diagnostician should be alert, or should attempt to provoke during a diagnostic interview.

Wilbur (quoted in Brandsma and Ludwig, 1974) has suggested the following four diagnostic signs:

1. Reports of time distortion or time lapses, including those called blackouts and spells by the patient.

2. Reports of being told of behavioral episodes by others which are not remembered by the patient.

3. Reports of notable changes in the patient's behaviour by a reliable observer, during which time the patient may call himself by different names or refer to himself in the third person.

4. Elicitability of other personalities through hypnosis.

To this list Greaves (1980) recommends that one adds a further four indicators:

5. The use of the word "we" in the course of an interview in which the word seems to take on a collective meaning other than the editorial "we".

6. The reported discovery of writings, drawings, or other productions or objects among the patient's belongings which he or she does not recognise and cannot account for.

7. A history of severe headaches, particularly when accompanied by blackouts, seizures, dreams, visions, visions, or deep sleeps.

8. The hearing of voices within a patient's head, entreating him or her to good or ill deeds, identified by the patient as originating from within but separate, and not

projected outward. (This latter addition was suggested by the work of Allison (1978).)

Thus despite a number of variations on the theme, the foregoing sample of definitions and descriptions from Taylor and Martin, Braun and Braun, DSM III, Wilbur, Greaves and Coons characterises what the American clinicians and researchers regard as the nature of multiple personality disorder. We shall see later that alternate personalities differ from each other, *inter alia*, in age, gender, sexual proclivities, handwriting styles, handedness, food preferences, response to medication, allergies, as well as in general attitudes, values and traits, such as interest in clothes and fashion, religiosity and social extraversion.

To complicate the picture a little there are sub-classifications of the syndrome. Ludwig et al. (1972), in a paper devoted to another of Dr Cornelia Wilbur's patients, Jonah, define multiple personality as;

> ... the presence of one or more alter personalities, each presumably (*sic*) possessing different sets of values and behaviours from one another and from the "primary" personality, and each claiming varying degrees of amnesia or disinterest for one another. The appearance of these alter personalities may be on a co-conscious basis (i.e. simultaneously coexistent with the primary personality and aware of its thoughts and feelings) or separate consciousness basis (i.e. alternating presence of the primary and alter personalities with little or no awareness or concern for the feelings and thoughts of each other), or both.

Ellenberger (1970), in his literary *tour de force*, *The Discovery of the Unconscious*, classifies the varieties of multiple personality syndrome as follows:

1. Simultaneous multiple personalities.
2. Succesive multiple personalities.
(a) mutually cognizant of each other.
(b) mutually amnesic.
(c) one-way amnesic.
3. Personality clusters.

Ellenberger calls "simultaneous multiple personalities" those cases where the disparate selves "are able to manifest themselves distinctly at one and the same moment." He states that these are rare, exceptional states and "Even when the two personalities are cognizant of each other, one of them is always dominant (even though the other's presence is being felt in the background)." He cites, by way of illustration, a patient of Bircher-Benner (1933) called "Ikara". At 15 this Zurich housewife suddenly felt convinced that, from personal experience, she knew about childbirth. Ten years on she became an in-patient and recounted vivid memories of previous existences, including living as a forest-dwelling primitive who ate the flesh of raw fowl. It seems that Dr Bircher-Benner took these reports as evidence of reincarnation and Ellenberger (1970), in delightful understatement, comments "It is regrettable that he (Bircher-Benner) did not make a detailed investigation of this patient's personal background." Perhaps one could be forgiven for not investing too much credence in evidence of this retrospective and incomplete nature.

As an example of "mutually cognizant personalities" Ellenberger cites a patient (Cory, 1920) where the one personality is described as cultured and inhibited whilst the alter ego is bold, passionate and speaks in broken Spanish. The latter, "personality B", was the dominant self and was supposed to be a spirit reincarnation. Allegedly, B was friendly with "a coterie of believers in spiritism who encourage her belief of being a returned spirit and over whom she exerts a tyrannical influence" (Ellenberger, 1970).

Such illustrations may be presented with Ellenberger's tongue firmly in cheek. Alternatively, they may lead to spiritualist phenomena being interpreted as further manifestations of multiple personality. Perhaps mediums are "honest liars", a phrase frequently used by Martin Orne to describe subjects who report, with sincere conviction, false memories implanted under hypnosis.

A much more famous character was Ansel Bourne whom William James (James, 1890) examined. Bourne, Ellenberger's illustration of his "mutually amnesic" category, was a religious convert who disappeared from home following a visit to his nephew. He then spent 2 months as a Pennsylvania shopkeeper under the alliterative pseudonym of Albert Brown. He had withdrawn money from his bank to finance the venture but seemingly had no recollection of his primary personality until he woke one morning, quite disorientated, and telephoned his nephew who came and brought him home. Only under hypnosis by James did Bourne recall his 2 months as Albert Brown but, with appropriate caution, Ellenberger writes "It is strange that in his secondary state, Albert Brown did not notice anything unusual about the papers, cheque book, and so on, bearing the name of Ansel Bourne, which he had with him all that time." Strange indeed; and disappointing that James does not tell us what may have led to his metamorphosis. It would appear that no further "switching" ever took place, and Bourne strikes one as an unlikely candidate for the diagnosis of multiple personality. Surely, "hysterical fugue state" would have been more appropriate and economical in this instance.

Most commonly reported in the literature on multiple personality are "one-way amnesics" and Ellenberger's illustrations are, once again, not the most convincing evidence. The cases are very dated and rest heavily on retrospective accounts. There is an absence of external corroboration of the patients' histories and the style of reporting is more journalistic than scientific. On this occasion we are introduced to two women, Felida (Azam, 1887), and Elena (Morselli, 1930). Parenthetically, one might note that Azam, unlike all the aforementioned commentators, was neither psychiatrist nor psychologist, but a professor of surgery at the Bordeaux Medical School. This aside is prompted by those who would suggest that multiple personality syndrome normally escapes the detection of the unspecialised eye. However, more about that later.

Felida was a polysymptomatic young woman whose hysterical symptoms would, almost daily, be followed by brief lethargy. She also suffered from panic attacks and hallucinations. Azam saw Felida when she presented with all the signs of pregnancy but was apparently oblivious to the fact that she had ever had intercourse. Following the diagnosis of pregnancy she shifted into her secondary personality and happily acknowledged her fecund state. She married and had ten more childbirths. During her life, her secondary (cheerful and healthy) personality was frequently to the fore and eventually became the norm. Felida must have been thankful for that since the primary personality that Azam describes was sickly indeed: "During her sleep, blood flowed slowly but continuously from her mouth. Any part of her body could suddenly become swollen, for instance, one half of her face" (Ellenberger, 1970). Although an allergic oedema might explain the swelling, such accounts certainly test one's credulity.

Morselli's patient, Elena, spoke in different languages when adopting her different personae. This 25-year-old piano teacher always believed herself to be speaking in Italian, her native tongue. However, her alter ego spoke in French, or sometimes in Italian-with-a French-accent. Elena knew nothing of her French persona. In common with Felida, Elena also suffered terrifying hallucinations but in contrast not only to Felida but to virtually all other recorded cases, her therapist judged the primary personality to be the more healthy. This is an intriguing issue with implications both for aetiology and treatment as we shall see later.

Whereas Felida never really recovered, constantly relapsing and haemorrhaging, Morselli was more successful with Elena. He interpreted her French condition as a denial of her father's existence (her father was an Italian-speaking native) because of incestuous assaults which she had repressed.

Ellenberger writes, "Most horrifying for her was the memory of his attempts to put his tongue into her mouth. Her flight into a French personality was thus an attempt to repress the memory of her father's 'tongue' and for his incestuous attacks in general" (Ellenberger, 1970). Abreactions helped her recover such memories and integrate her two personalities.

Morselli was quite an adventurous researcher, taking mescalin and reporting that he was metamorphosing into a werewolf.

Finally, Ellenberger notes that although the early accounts of multiple personality were dual-personalities so strikingly embodied in Dr Jekyll and Mr Hyde, there have been frequent reports of more than two selves inhabiting the same body, which he terms "personality clusters". He cites the example of Miss Beauchamp whose case was well documented by Morton Prince in his monograph, *The Dissociation of a Personality* (1906). Prince saw Miss Beauchamp when she was 23 and complaining of headaches, lassitude and fatiguability. Under hypnosis two further personalities emerged; the one was Miss Beauchamp writ large (conscientious, introverted and scholarly) whilst the other was extraverted and rebellious. Prince referred to these personalities as B1, B2, and B3, and the amnestic network was as follows: B1 knew nothing about the existence of B2 or B3; B3 knew all about B1 and B2; B2 knew only about B1 but not about B3. To complicate matters a little further, a fourth, regressive personality was to appear; but we have already encountered more recent cases, Eve and Sybil, where 22 and 16 personalities have been reported. Notwithstanding, the record must surely go to the patient of Dr Eugene Bliss, only the third multiple personality patient he had ever diagnosed. He describes her as "a classical hysteric with a multiplicity of somatic symptoms and a long list of major surgical operations. She had never been perceived as multiple, and none in her family had recognised distinct characters. None the less I tried hypnosis, which opened Pandora's box. Out came a host of personalities, with names and functions–at last count almost fifty" (Bliss, 1986, pp. 120–121). Presumably, it is to this patient that Coons (1980) was referring earlier.

Here Bliss clearly illustrates how a psychiatrist who has seen (or, at least, recognised) only two previous multiple personality patients can go on to uncover in one individual more than fifty latent selves "almost by accident" (*sic*); the most dramatic count of all provoked by a self-confessed novice who, in this instance, had no reason at all to suspect the presence of this exotic syndrome.

Bliss (1986) prefaces his book, *Multiple Personality, Allied Disorders, and Hypnosis*, with a résumé of his encounter with his first multiple personality patient. She was a nurse called Sarah. A chief nurse, suspecting that Sarah was abusing a morphine analogue, Demerol, had called Sarah into her office and exposed the tell-tale needle marks on her arms. At this point, Sarah metamorphosed into a bewildered and tearful "Sue". (Bliss's original reference to this nurse appears some years earlier (Bliss, 1980) when he wrote "she claimed her name was not Lois but Jane." This inconsistency in detail is not uncommon in the multiple personality literature as will become evident). Bliss tells us that he immediately accepted the referral because he suspected a case of multiple personality. He goes on, "It became apparent that the reason I had never seen a case in the past 30 years of psychiatric practice as an academician–a teacher, investigator, and therapist–was simply ignorance. Many such patients must have escaped my detection over the years as they passed through the psychiatric service" (Bliss, 1986).

However, Dr Bliss's confession of ignorance is surely inappropriate modesty. Sarah/Sue (or Lois/Jane) revealed her alter ego at the outset, the sole provocation being her exposure by a senior nurse. The absence of such self-disclosure in Bliss's previous patients could be explained more economically by assuming they were not suffering from multiple personalities.

Notwithstanding, having identified Sarah as the first case he had seen over a span of 30 years (knowingly, at any rate), Bliss goes on to inform us that "Astonishingly, another case was identified by a resident in the emergency room a few weeks later" (Bliss, 1986). This patient had eighteen identified and named personalities. Yet again, we have a graphic illustration of a relatively inexperienced doctor, the resident, recognising multiple personality.

It is customary, and helpful, when presenting an illness syndrome to provide some information about incidence (the rate of new cases over a specified period, usually a year), and prevalence (the frequency of all cases at a particular time). Stable rates of incidence and prevalence are proportional, so that at any one time: prevalence = incidence/duration of illness.

It must be already apparent that there are insufficient reliable data about incidence and prevalence apropos of multiple personality. However, this is not to say that the therapists and writers in this area have not proffered a few estimates based on their personal experiences.

Coons (1984) writes "I personally know of ten multiple personality cases in the Indianapolis metropolitan area with a population of 1 million. Therefore, an incidence of 1 to 100,000 would be a conservative estimate."

The research report of Bliss and Jeppsen (1985) would indicate that this was a very conservative estimate. Addressing themselves to the issue of prevalence they conducted a survey of psychiatric inpatients and outpatients which led the authors to conclude that of their 150 patient sample "Approximately 10% had multiple personality." They found no significant difference between inpatients sequentially admitted to two acute wards of a university hospital (N = 50), and two series (N = 100) randomly drawn from the files of a psychiatrist in private practice with routine referrals "from diverse sources".

Kluft (1984) has reported that "Over a decade I interviewed 171 MPD [multiple personality disorder] patients from my own practice and research ... [and] one hundred and seventeen patients with clearly defined classic MPD sought treatment with me."

Horevitz and Braun (1984), in the same symposium, say they had access to the case notes of 93 patients with this diagnosis "interviewed since 1977".

Bliss (1984) seems to summarise the current view of such psychiatrists when he writes: "The implication is that cases of multiple personalities are rare. This is the general belief, although it is probably incorrect. Cases are now being detected in large numbers and I have personally seen 100 in the last 4 years. If my experience is representative, these cases are relatively common ...."

However, this author wrote to the Bulletins of the British Psychological Society, and of the Royal College of Psychiatrists, at the beginning of 1987, to canvass whether British colleagues had any comparable experience. Given that the joint readership of these two publications runs into many thousands it was surprising that only a handful of replies were received. Of these, only four came from psychopathologists who believed they might have seen such patients (a total of six between them), and all were couched in the most tentative terms.

If such evidence were necessary, it is clear that some therapists have an astronomically higher probability of meeting such patients than their colleagues and the vast majority (dare one say, "all"?)are in the United States. Such a significant epidemiological difference cries out for explanation.

Could it be that one's American colleagues are quite simply more skilful diagnosticians of this syndrome? Such a generous view is certainly not shared by Tony Armond, a consultant psychiatrist from Birmingham, England. I quote in full his reply to my Bulletin letter:

"In the UK, we react to any suggestion by patients or relatives that there are two or more personalities by immediately saying that there are two or more aspects to one personality, and asserting that the individual must take responsibility for both of these aspects. It works.

In the USA there has been interest in, and a history of much money being made of, multiple personality as a concept. The patient can be led into confirming the keen enquirer's expectations; and sustaining the system of beliefs can become a hobby for both. The danger is that the patient indulges in deplorable behaviour and absolves himself, or more usually, herself, from responsibility for it.

I had one patient who sustained the belief that he had several named personalities and behaved as if he totally believed it. You may be disappointed to know that Modecate restored him to his former unitary self and removed other delusional beliefs, for he was psychotic."

One could not ask for a more definitive response, so is the whole business a myth? Does this extensively documented Emperor have fewer vestments than his devotees imagine? Are gullible psychiatrists being taken for a ride by a group of manipulative patients who want licence for their deviant behaviour? Or are gullible patients being taken for a ride by psychiatrists seeking financial and/or personal aggrandisement? Such *ad hominem* argument apart, could a vast number of highly qualified and respected clinician-researchers, of undoubted integrity, be radically wrong?

The ensuing chapters will present and evaluate the protean evidence that has been adduced to support the thesis that multiple personality syndrome exists as a discrete clinical entity. It will already be apparent that this thesis rests on surer foundations than the antiquated reports of questionable validity collated by Professor Ellenberger.

How much surer must be left to the reader to decide for there are many positions to occupy along the spectrum between credulity and scepticism, positions which will doubtless shift as the evidence unfolds. In the chapters that follow there is a welter of evidence to be weighed and sifted before drawing any conclusions and it will quickly be appreciated that the problem is as multi-faceted as the phenomenon that it purports to underlie.

CHAPTER 2

The Case of the Hillside Strangler

This chapter is devoted to the case of Kenneth Bianchi, aged 27, who was arrested in January, 1979, charged with the murder of two college girls. Eight other young women had been raped and strangled and the naked bodies of some had been displayed on hillsides in the Los Angeles, earning the murderer the lurid name of "The Hillside Strangler." The case graphically illustrates the difficulties in diagnosing multiple personality even when (or perhaps, especially when) a plethora of experts is involved. I have stuck closely to my principal sources, three papers (Watkins, 1984; Allison, 1984; Orne, Dinges and Orne, 1984) which appear together in the April, 1984, issue of the *International Journal of Clinical and Experimental Hypnosis* which focused on multiple personality.

The first paper is by Dr John Watkins, a noted authority, who has been involved in the evaluation and treatment of multiple personality since 1946, and who runs training courses on hypnosis and multiple personality with his wife, Helen, in Laguna Beach, California. Despite damning circumstantial evidence that Bianchi was guilty of the two crimes he insisted he had no recollection of the significant portion of the night in question. Dean Brett, his lawyer, called in John Watkins to see if hypnosis could recover his memories for this night as well, perhaps, as for other periods of "blanking-out" which he reported.

Watkins was impressed that Bianchi did not want to enter an insanity plea and that he presented as a mild and pleasant young man whose history contraindicated the diagnosis of sociopathic personality disorder. He also seemed unconcerned for his legal fate but instead was preoccupied with understanding himself better. He had been a nervous child with tics, allergies, incontinence, petit mal episodes, and numerous phobias. His mother, however, resisted explanations from the many professionals he saw that these symptoms had an emotional basis. Although Bianchi professed loyalty and respect for his mother she was both seductive (showing him nude pictures) and cruel (holding his hand over the cooker and beating him with a belt). Bianchi's common-law wife said he was a good husband and father to their small child.

At first, Bianchi was fearful of being hypnotised but Watkins persevered and eventually induced a substantially deep trance. He then gave a suggestion to Bianchi which he knew had been effective in "breaking through an amnesia, activating a covert ego state or inducing a multiple personality to become overt." The suggestion was:

I've talked a bit to Ken, but I think that perhaps there might be another part of Ken that I haven't talked to, another part that maybe feels somewhat differently from the part I've talked to. And I would like to communicate with that other part.

Watkins stresses that he did not cue the content of this part.

Bianchi responded by saying that he was not Ken but someone called Steve who, in fact, hated Ken because "he tries to be nice." He also said he hated his mother and went on to relate how Ken had walked in on his cousin, Angelo Buono, when he was "killing this girl." He confessed that he (Steve) had strangled and killed "all these girls", adding "I fixed him (Ken) up good. He doesn't even have any idea." Steve elaborated on the details of the killings and then Ken was brought back, still under hypnosis, but he denied all knowledge of Steve and was amnesic for all that had just transpired when he came out of his trance.

Watkins insists (in a footnote) that neither Bianchi nor his lawyer knew that he was a specialist in multiple personality prior to their first meeting.

On the following day Watkins "reactivated" Steve who provided more details about how he kept knowledge of his existence from Ken. He also states that he asked whether there were any other personalities and "Bill" was mentioned but, for reasons Watkins does not explain, "I did not activate and explore this personality."

Steve recounted childhood incidents when he had "come out", misbehaved, and then left Ken to cope. "I let him come back again, and sit there and think about it. Stupid ass-hole." He said that Ken had no hint of his presence; "Fuck no, it would ruin me ... he's not aware ... that I am what I am."

He also seemed to be unaware that what happened to Ken also would happen to him when he showed a callous disregard for Ken's future: "I hope they fucking roast him ... he would be out of my hair." Watkins observes that such logical inconsistency typifies both multiple personality patients and deeply hypnotised subjects.

His conviction that he was dealing with a multiple personality patient rather than hypnotic artefact is evidenced when he writes, "The two personalities behaved differently in almost every respect: manner, attitude, language, posture, gestures, speech, behaviours, values."

At this stage, the court appointed six experts to examine the 65 hours of audio- and video-tapes, and Watkins was asked to return a month later. He decided that a diagnosis of multiple personality would be determined if Steve could be activated without hypnosis and if psychological test data were available for both personalities. Watkins especially favoured using the Rorschach which he says is " most difficult to fake" whilst providing no empirical support for this assertion. One might venture that the Rorschach inkblot test, and projective tests in general, are not without their distinguished critics. More will said about the inadequacies of such techniques in Chapter 4 but Professor Philip Vernon, international expert on personality assessment, wrote (Vernon, 1964, p. 175), "(projective techniques) are not worth using unless they yield information which cannot be obtained by ordinary case-history methods and tests such as MMPI. The evidence at present available suggests that they detract from, rather than add to, such methods."

At his second interview, Watkins avoided hypnosis but Ken was already referring to Steve and his "readiness to fight." This was attributable to Ken having seen Dr Ralph Allison in the interim. Allison is an equally distinguished specialist in multiple personality and had seen Ken "for several days" in the month that intervened between Watkins' first and second interviews with Bianchi. During these sessions, Allison had hypnotised Bianchi and "introduced" Steve and Ken to each other. (Watkins acknowledged this as a mistake which hampered differential diagnosis). Ken said he felt unwell which Watkins surmised was evidence of a secondary personality trying to emerge. He states, "I focused on this point and asked him repeatedly why he felt bad. With an angry snarl, Steve emerged voicing his dislike of me and loudly complaining of his difficulty in getting out now that Ken knew about his existence." This is a curious complaint since Watkins is telling us that Steve emerged to no more prompting than enquiry as to why Ken felt unwell.

Watkins reports that he then gave the Rorschach to Steve but first showed him magazine pictures of girl victims of the "Hillside Strangler." Steve was co-operative, even excited, and pointed out those whom he had killed, together with those murdered by his cousin, Buono. Watkins says he did this to win Steve's co-operation but he must be aware that it may well have created a particular mental set for the Rorschach which was administered immediately afterwards.

Following this, "Ken was reactivated ... feeling that he had been "asleep" for only a few minutes." Watkins does not say how this reactivation took place but it is implicit that deliberate hypnosis was not employed.

The resultant protocols were sent for blind appraisal to two Rorschach experts, Dr Richard Ball (formerly of the Albert Einstein Medical School) and Professor Erika Fromm (from the University of Chicago, and clinical editor of the *International Journal of Clinical and Experimental Hypnosis*). Fromm did not recognise that the records were from the same individual and said that Ken's Rorschach was within normal limits, if mildly neurotic. (This, of course, is quite remarkable when one recalls Ken as a boy who was riddled with phobic fears and nervous twitches and had a seductive sadist for a mother.) Steve's protocol, however, was interpreted most impressively as that of a dangerous and violent person. Fromm wrote, "I would expect him to be a rapist and a killer." She goes on to say that "he is not a psychopath; he could be a schizophrenic ...."

Dr Ball diagnosed Ken as follows: "There does not appear to be any clear evidence of (1) low intelligence, (2) psychopathic personality, (3) organic brain impairment, (4) psychotic process either affective or schizoid. I lean toward a diagnosis of hysterical neurosis, dissociative type." His summary diagnosis of Steve was "Sadism". Ball was told that both Rorschachs came from one man, and Ball opined that there was no evidence of malingering.

Watkins also provides us with the opinion of a Rorschach expert secured by Dr Martin Orne. This Rorschacher thought the protocol (Watkins does not say which one) did indicate psychopathy and not multiple personality. She reported a "Delta Index" (Watkins and Stauffacher, 1952) of 0% for both Ken and Steve. Watkins informs us that this index purports to be "a measure of the extent to which primitive, concrete (psychotic) ideation has invaded reality testing." He disagrees with her scoring and states that, "Ken did score 0%, but Steve's Delta should have scored 25% – clearly, within the psychotic range." It will be obvious already why so many contemporary psychologists have such little faith in Rorschach scores.

Dr Edwin Wagner, erroneously cited by Watkins as the sole publisher of a paper on Rorschach responses and multiple personality (see, for example, Danesino et al., 1979), also saw the protocols but did not think that Bianchi was a case either of multiple personality or psychopathy.

Watkins goes on to tell us that the MMPI "was given to Ken, but not to Steve." Why this procedure was adopted is a mystery. Just three pages earlier Watkins had explained that the rationale for using psychological tests was that they "should be administered separately to Steve and Ken." Given that there are no MMPI norms for multiple personality it is hard to understand why it was given to Ken here.

As further evidence to support his diagnosis of multiple personality we learn that a graphologist asked to comment on the handwriting of Ken and Steve, together with two other "personalities" who apparently had emerged. However, the analysis was not blind and was made many months after the case was closed. Watkins is the first to point out this fundamental weakness and one assumes that courtesy rather than scientific curiosity led him to allow this graphologist to demonstrate her prowess (she was the wife of a psychology colleague). In the event her descriptions of Ken and Steve were predictably different and she declared the handwriting styles appeared to belong to different authors.

We are told that further evidence is Ken's preference for filter-tips (Steve tears them off), his high school sculpture of a two-faced head and sketches in jail of fragmented human figures.

Watkins also relates Bianchi's reported instances of amnesia over many years. Even though he admits that these could not be corroborated his faith in his diagnosis is unshakable; "patients suffering from amnesic episodes often conceal them from others to avoid embarrassment", writes Watkins.

A Dr Lunde is quoted as saying that Bianchi was neither "psychologically sophisticated enough nor ... intelligent enough" to have been faking. I must be allowed to disagree. Watkins himself informs us that Bianchi had posed as a psychologist, albeit briefly, and a number of psychology books were found at his home, albeit of a popular rather than scholarly nature. As for his intelligence, Watkins says his WAIS IQ was

116; in Wechsler's words "bright-normal" and lying well within the top 15% of the population. How bright does one have to be to feign mental illness?

Watkins even argues that Bianchi's use of the passive tense is yet more evidence of multiple personality as when he said "the girls were strangled" rather than "I strangled the girls." This Watkins interprets as the lack of involvement of Bianchi's self, and indicative of dissociative defences.

In October, 1979, Bianchi finally admitted to the crimes, carried out with his cousin Buono. He pled guilty to 7 murders and was sentenced to life imprisonment. Watkins, however, expresses what happened thus: "By October, 1979, Ken had become 'convinced' that 'he' had actually committed the crimes." Ironically, Watkins is suggesting that Bianchi was brainwashed out of his multiple personality state and ended up feigning the sociopath. Since Bianchi has been in prison he has again taken to denying all knowledge of the murders.

Martin Orne is quoted as not believing that Bianchi was ever hypnotised, either by himself, Watkins or Allison (the only experts to use hypnotic induction with Bianchi). Orne carried out a number of "objective tests" under hypnosis which he judged Bianchi failed but Watkins exposes the subjective nature of these tests by challenging Orne's interpretation at every turn. For example, Orne suggested to Bianchi that he hallucinate his lawyer seated opposite him. His lawyer was in fact behind him. Bianchi obliged by "seeing" his lawyer seated opposite and was then confronted with the real lawyer behind him. Orne argues that at this point genuinely hypnotised subjects (reals allegedly) exhibit "trance logic" whereby they calmly accept the incongruous experience. Bianchi failed because he expressed undue concern and surprise. Although Watkins has earlier described Orne as "perhaps the world authority on the danger of possible simulation" he now dismisses Orne's opinion out of hand. "The qualification that visualisation of the two images... must be accompanied by a lack of concern is definitely not a valid criterion." Similarly, Orne argues that reals see hallucinated images as transparent whereas Bianchi said the image was like that under a strobe light ("little bits and pieces"). Could this not be the same as "transparent", asks Watkins? And is it not further confirmation that Bianchi carried on talking with the hallucination when Orne left the room?

The more cynical might argue that prisoners under rigorous investigation take it for granted that they are always under surveillance whether using sophisticated bugging devices and cameras or a simple hole in the wall. Watkins also refers to Orne's use of the circle-touch test which again focuses on trance-logic. A circle is drawn on the subject's arm and s/he is told to say "Yes" when touched outside the circle, and "No" when touched inside the circle because here there will be no feeling. Simulators spot the contradiction and say nothing when touched inside the hypnotically anaesthetised area. Reals, however, respond with "No." Unfortunately, the first time that Orne administered the circle-touch test his back obscured the camera so we cannot know which stimuli produced the responses. However, the presence of a single "No" response leads Watkins to say that Bianchi was a "real." On the second, unobscured, administration all touches inside the circle (4) produced no response and, reasonably enough, Orne concludes that Bianchi was simulating. Watkins, however, argues that no response could indicate a genuine lack of sensation and Orne failed to check on this. Watkins also criticises Orne for using a pen-point rather than a Von Frey hair to control for equal pressure, and for failing to allow a minimum of 4 seconds between trials (Orne allowed an average 2.3 seconds). If a subject is not given sufficient time, Watkins argues, their absence of response may simply indicate a delayed reaction. Finally, Orne employed the "source-amnesia" test. Here subjects are given obscure bits of knowledge under hypnosis (e.g. that amethysts turn yellow when heated) and are wakened with suggestions of amnesia. Later when asked, say, about the colour of heated amethysts they will give the right answer but will be unable to identify the source of their knowledge. In the event, Bianchi said he did not know the answer to the amethyst question. When asked about the capital of Arkansas (he had been taught "Little Rock" under hypnosis) Bianchi gave the right answer but attributed the source to a song title. Confusion reigns and Watkins is right to be critical of Orne.

It is not so much Bianchi who fails on this and the previous "objective" items but that the items themselves fail. The clumsiness of administration, the paucity of trials, the absence of controls, the subjective nature of ascribing "pass" or "fail" to performances, the absence of consensus amongst the experts as to what responses characterise "reals" as opposed to simulators, render Orne's test battery largely worthless which is as disappointing as it is surprising given Orne's international status as fake-detector. These results do not help us to decide whether Bianchi was faking hypnosis. Furthermore, to quote Watkins, "whether he was hypnotised or not is irrelevant to the diagnosis since true multiple personalities emerge without hypnosis." In fairness to Orne, however, if it had been proved that Bianchi was a fake when it came to being hypnotised it would surely have been further evidence that his multiple personality performance was similarly bogus.

Allison (1984) had seen 49 patients diagnosed as multiple personality in the 7 years before he met Bianchi in 1979. Like Watkins, he can claim to be an internationally acclaimed expert. Unlike Watkins, he began by diagnosing Bianchi as a multiple personality but then changed his mind in favour of an atypical dissociative disorder caused by the examining methods themselves!

Allison saw Bianchi for two 1-day sessions in the April and June. After an initial interview he was age-regressed to 9, 13 and then when he reached 27, Steve appeared. Steve was crude, aggressive and foul mouthed and readily admitted to multiple murder. He denied any other personalities "inside" Ken. Allison asked Ken, under hypnosis, to conduct a "telephone conversation" with Steve. He writes, "Ken appeared to know Steve, accept his existence, and know that Steve ... had committed the murders." This is in stark contrast to Watkins' impression of Bianchi. Watkins not only asserts unequivocally that Ken knew nothing of Steve ("Who's Steve?" he had asked when out of hypnosis) but further, that it was Allison who was responsible for Ken's awareness of his murderous alter-ego. Watkins wrote, "Dr Allison had seen Ken for several days (in fact only 1½ days) and was convinced he was a genuine multiple personality (curiously, Watkins fails to report that Allison later changed his diagnosis).

He had "introduced Ken to Steve under hypnosis ... Ken knew now of the existence of Steve."

From the videotape of Orne's session with Bianchi, Allison learned of two other putative personalities, a 9-year-old Ken who cried, and a 14-year-old larcenist called Billy. In June, Allison set out to interview Billy beginning with Bianchi's "inner self-helper" or "Ken's friend" as it called itself. Handwriting samples were obtained, Billy and Steve emerged to take the California Personality Inventory (separately, that is) and this test was left with Bianchi's social worker so that Ken could complete it later. Bianchi had already completed the CPI and the MMPI back in April. Ken also used the Identi-Kit to make faces of Billy and Steve.

Allison seems to have had little difficulty in hypnotising Bianchi and talking to all the personalities and getting them to complete the tests. They told him it was Billy who posed as the psychologist (but using the name Thomas Steven Walker) and that Bianchi had been infected with gonorrhoea by his wife who said she had been raped on holiday. The "inner self-helper" said this weakened Bianchi and allowed Steve to "come out".

The psychological test results are not the most illuminating. Ken's April MMPI indicated hysterical dissociation. His CPI produced the preferred diagnosis of personality disorder and possible drink problem. In June the personality disorder was still indicated together with paranoid and passive-aggressive elements. Billy's June CPI also indicated a personality disorder of the dissociative type. Steve's June CPI indicated paranoid schizophrenia. Allison makes no further comment concerning these results. No discussion follows their presentation. No conclusions are drawn. No rationale for their administration is given.

Regarding the Identi-Kit pictures Allison reports only that neither picture looked like Bianchi and he adds the cryptic comment that "both matched the personality characteristics seen on interview." Could Allison be suggesting in some post-Lombrosian manner that our faces reflect our personality?

Eventually, Allison submitted a 124-page report to the court concluding that Bianchi was insane by reason of multiple personality syndrome but, as we now know, the court rejected that submission and Allison was to change his mind.

This change of mind was revealed during the trial, 2 years later, of Bianchi's cousin, Buono. Allison reports that after reviewing the transcripts "the facts which I now looked at with more attention fitted a dissociative disorder, but not what I knew to be the multiple personality syndrome." He continues by asserting that the personalities "Steve," "Billy," and "Ken's Friend" were iatrogenically created by Watkins, Orne and himself, respectively. He then lists 17 reasons for his change of diagnosis which I summarise as follows:

1. Ken was able to express the full range of emotions unlike multiple personality patients where such expression has been inhibited and de facto given rise to the birth of alter egos who can express these feelings.

2. Steve was not mentioned until Allison mooted the idea of "hiding in his own head" having regressed Bianchi to age 9.

3. Steve allegedly first emerged while Bianchi was hiding under a bed whereas alter egos normally appear in response to a specific trauma.

4. Bianchi had a best friend living next door whereas multiple personality patients are typically lonely as children with no confidants.

5. Instead of Steve having a different attitude to school from Ken, which one would expect from an alter ego, both disliked it equally.

6. Bianchi reported having many friends but if Steve had really existed when Bianchi was a child he would surely have repelled them.

7. When regressed to age 13, the alleged time of the creation of Billy at his father's death, Bianchi did not refer to his bereavement without prompting. Should not such a significant crisis have been mentioned at once by Bianchi?

8. Billy was supposed to have been created following repeated visits to his father's coffin whereas one would have expected an alter ego to emerge when he first learned of his father's death. In fact, he took the tragic news relatively well.

9. Unlike the victims of other murderers with multiple personality syndrome seen by Allison, those of Bianchi had no emotional tie to him nor did they constitute any personal threat.

10. Bianchi showed atypical fatigue after switching personalities.

11. When asked to carry on a "telephone conversation" with Steve, Bianchi co-operated too literally unlike any of Allison's multiple personality patients. Also highly atypical was Bianchi's reported amnesia for this internal dialogue.

12. When asked about the presence of other personalities besides Steve, Bianchi signalled that there were none. Either he was lying, because Billy was already present, or Billy did not emerge until Orne challenged Steve as being an adequate explanation for the pose as a professional psychologist.

13. The fact that Bianchi did not need dehypnotising after the age regression and emergence of Steve makes Allison question whether he was ever hypnotised in the first place.

14. Criminals with multiple personalities do not accuse others of their crimes. In a letter to Allison, after the trial, Bianchi accused a man called Greg but police investigations failed to corroborate his allegations.

15. Bianchi enlisted the aid of a woman who posted a tape to Allison with a recording of a man "confessing" to Bianchi's crimes and to having framed him. When arrested (for the attempted murder of a woman in a motel room) more tapes were found in her possession with recorded threats to Allison's daughters. Allison says that such hostility towards their therapist is unknown amongst genuine multiple personality ex-patients.

16. Bianchi was a self-confessed chronic liar. "Lying" amongst multiple personality patients normally results from their ignorance of acts carried out by alternate personalities.

17. None has ever witnessed any of the personality changes; family, friends or prison staff.

Allison concludes that Bianchi was not deliberately faking but that he was suffering from an atypical dissociative disorder (DSM III, p.260) "occurring under stress of intensive and extensive psychiatric evaluations, while under threat of the death penalty, and limited in duration to the period of time between arrests for murder and sentencing."

Orne, Dinges and Orne (1984), however, argue that Bianchi was a sexually sadistic psychopath deliberating simulating multiple personality to avoid the death penalty. The main thrust of the paper is whether or not individuals can successfully fake this syndrome and, given their conclusion, the answer would seem to be a resounding "Yes" although Bianchi clearly did not deceive Orne.

A large number of factors led Orne to his sceptical conclusion including performance on some of his procedures to distinguish real from feigned hypnosis although some doubt has already been cast on the validity of this battery. For example, Orne observed that when Bianchi was asked to hallucinate his lawyer and then confronted with the real person, he "overacted" showing great puzzlement and asking persistently, "How can Dean Brett (his lawyer) be in two places?" Orne says that the "double hallucination" procedure in "reals" leads to a *belle indifférence*. Similarly, when Bianchi was asked to hallucinate his lawyer sitting opposite him and to converse with him, Bianchi responded by leaning forward and "shaking the hand" of the hallucination. He went on to involve Orne, saying, "So what's going on? What we gonna talk about, the three of us?" Also, he insisted to Orne that he "must be able to see him." Orne asserts that these three aspects of his performance do not characterise the behaviour of genuinely hypnotised subjects.

Orne acknowledges that the source amnesia and circle touch tests did not discriminate between hypnosis and simulation.

Bianchi repeatedly expressed great surprise when, having "returned" as Ken, he was confronted with evidence of Steve's recent presence. For example, it has already been remarked that Steve preferred to remove the tips from filter cigarettes. When Steve was "out" he would smoke several cigarettes leaving behind a conspicuous pile of filters. On Ken's "return" he would express amazement at the pile of filters and ask how they got there. Orne rightly suggests that after this had happened for the first time, and Bianchi had been informed that it was Steve's doing, he would surely not keep on being amazed and keep on seeking explanations as he did from Watkins, Allison and Orne. A more likely explanation is that Bianchi was putting on exaggerated performances of his amnesia for each expert in turn.

When it comes to the personalities themselves, Orne makes a number of telling points. Firstly, there was a lack of consistency in the personality of Steve. When he first emerged, before Watkins, "his behaviour at this time, however, was not threatening, he spoke in a low voice, frequently laughed mockingly, did not curse, was relatively polite, made no demands and was motorically passive." On the next occasion, Steve had begun to curse, and was more animated and aggressive. By the time Allison saw him, Steve had become loud, coarse, agitated and threatening, "a caricature of a macho man." This picture conflicts with the notion of a well-formed and integrated personality existing since the age of 9. Further, when asked if Steve had a surname, he replied "Walker", and it will be remembered that it was in the name of

Thomas Steven Walker that Bianchi had arrogated forged psychology diplomas. Investigations revealed that Steven Walker really existed but only came to Bianchi's attention in 1978. In order to obtain false diplomas Bianchi had posed as a psychologist and advertised for a colleague to join his practice. Thomas Steven Walker MA was one of many applicants who sent Bianchi his transcripts as part of his application. Bianchi then wrote to Walker's college, pretending to be Walker, saying he had lost his diplomas, and could the college send him duplicates. He added that he did not want his name filled in because he was employing a calligrapher for this purpose to enter his name in elaborate script. Amazingly, the college complied with this request. Clearly, unless one stretches ones' imagination to the ultimate, Bianchi knew of no Steven Walker until the time that his initial murders were being committed. It is highly improbable that he had a boyhood friend of just the same name who acted as inspiration for the identity of his alleged alter ego, supposedly emerging 18 years previously, when he was only 9 years old. What is also abundantly apparent is that Bianchi was a very clever character, devising an ingenious set of tactics to acquire his false credentials.

In addition to the questionable nature of the Steve alter ego that Bianchi produced is the question of the number of personalities. Orne tells us that until he saw him only one alternate, Steve, had emerged. Suspecting a fraud, Orne put it to Bianchi that multiple personality patients typically manifested at least three personalities. Almost immediately,"a new personality emerged, and responded that it needed more time before coming out. It said its name was 'Billy,' and he agreed to come out during the next session; which would be before dinner." Orne concluded that Bianchi's readiness to produce personalities on cue, coupled with Bianchi actually allowing himself time to perfect the role they might play, could only call into further question the validity of the diagnosis of multiple personality syndrome.

As well as reiterating Allison's point that there was no external corroboration for Bianchi's alleged personality switches, Orne reveals that the boyhood sculpture of Bianchi, the Janus figure which Watkins felt was so clinically significant, was the product of two individuals! Apparently, Bianchi told Dr Lunde that (in Orne's words) "the two heads were an 'accident' in that [he] had difficulty in forming the back of the head and it therefore became a joint project wherein another student sculpted the ape's face!"

In the matter of the psychological test data, Orne makes the astute observation that blind diagnosticians, when presented with several test protocols, will take it for granted that they come from different individuals. Given that a multiple personality is, to say the least, an unlikely initial hypothesis, one could forgive the most expert diagnostician for assuming that two Rorschachs or two MMPIs come from two individuals, especially when they are so labelled by a professional colleague. Thus the initial mental set of the blind diagnostician, whatever the outcome of the analyses of content or profile, is that one is dealing with as many individuals as there are proforma. It is psychologically naive to argue that multiple personality is in evidence because the blind evaluator concludes that two sets of test data indicate two different respondents.

Orne decided to ask a more appropriate and sophisticated question of his blind evaluator, Dr Margaret Singer; "whether the Rorschach records reflected different personalities that are essentially autonomous, or whether they did not." Singer's reply was clear enough; "I regard these two records to be simply reflections of one man, who is a sociopathic personality." She notes that on the first record (as Ken) Bianchi treats the tester "politely" whereas the second record (as Steve) indicates role enactment as someone who was "irritable, rude [and] uncooperative." Underlying these superficial differences, however, Singer points to strikingly similar "thought, attention and associative properties." Orne et al. note that Wagner drew a similar conclusion which has been cited earlier in this chapter.

Dr Harrison Gough was asked to look at the CPI profiles for Ken, Steve and Billy, in the full knowledge that it was Bianchi who had produced all three proformas. Gough concluded that "the three personalities ... do not seem to be three distinct and different individuals, but rather roles or variations developed from a common core."

There are fundamental problems concerning the appropriateness of giving psychological tests to putative multiple personalities. Firstly, there is the problem of the objectivity of the evaluator. If the evaluator is told that the records come from a single individual they are set to perceive common characteristics. If the evaluator is told nothing, but simply given several proformas they will naturally assume that they come from as many individuals and will be set to focus on differences between the sets of data. Secondly, the tests can hardly be used diagnostically since no norms exist for multiple personality populations. Thirdly, there is an absence of control group data in that, as Orne et al. note, "research is needed to determine how well clinicians can distinguish between test data derived from authenticated multiple personality cases, versus data from individuals role-playing or faking multiplicity, versus records from different individuals submitted as though they were obtained from a suspected multiple personality."

With regard to how easily the expert can be fooled, it is salutary to attend to Orne's studies of simulation carried out in 1960. Orne had Milton Erikson, pre-eminent amongst hypnotists, try to distinguish simulators from deeply hypnotised subjects but despite Erikson's experience with thousands of subjects and, what Orne terms his "undisputed mastery of the field," he was unable to do so. Paradoxically, however, Orne infers that he (or someone) could make such discriminations, if only on a probabilistic basis, for someone must have identified the criterion groups against which Erikson's performance was assessed! Nonetheless, one hopes Orne has finally laid the ghost that only the most gifted actor is capable of simulating multiple personality to the point where an expert can be fooled.

Orne goes on to discuss whether it would have been helpful in Bianchi's case to adopt less stringent criteria for the presence of multiple personality syndrome. Gruenewald (1977a,b) has suggested that "the symptomatology of multiple personalities lies on a continuum from mild and/or transient to severe and/or long lasting." From the perspective of ego-state theory, Watkins (1976) argues that personality comprises a number of ego-states with more or less permeable boundaries. Watkins further suggests that, in good hypnotic subjects, such ego-states may "become" pseudo-alternate personalities following hypnotic intervention. However, Orne makes the point that the adoption of increasingly less stringent criteria in line with such a concept of a continuum of multiple personality syndrome makes "the possibility of ever falsifying the diagnosis ... increasingly tenuous."

Finally, though not directly relevant to the diagnosis of multiple personality, is the issue of Bianchi's insanity at the time he committed the murders. Orne summarises that the crimes evidenced careful planning and premeditation, that the motive was straightforward sexual lust, that there was no evidence of thought disorder or psychosis, and that Bianchi strenuously avoided being apprehended. One might add that even after conviction Bianchi continued to conspire to lay the blame for the crimes elsewhere. (He even wrote to his mother asking her to type an anonymous confession to be sent to the *Seattle Times*. However, his mother refused, preferring to inform his lawyer of this request.) Interestingly, Allison (1984) had concluded, "I believe that he [Bianchi] also unconsciously set himself up to be caught ... so that he could be stopped forever." Hypotheses resting on the foundations of unconscious motivation are not, of course, falsifiable.

The case of The Hillside Strangler highlights the enormous problems in diagnosing multiple personality even when a vast amount of biographical and videotape data are available, and internationally renowned experts are involved in hundreds of hours of diagnostic examination. Also brought into focus is the value or otherwise of psychological testing in this context, and the absence of objective criteria for both the presence of a true hypnotic trance and multiple personality syndrome. In the forensic setting, where the secondary gain for simulation can be a matter of life or death, the problems surrounding differential diagnosis are all the more exacerbated.

However, despite the final judgement of the court in line with the majority expert opinion, there will always remain those clinicians, like Dr Watkins, who remain convinced that Bianchi really was a case of multiple personality.

CHAPTER 3

The Voice of the Sceptics

It is not unknown for psychiatry to be in dissent. Although rather passé, Laing lingers on and there are doubtless acolytes still who would insist that schizophrenia does not exist (not quite what Laing said, of course). Similarly, following the lead of Szasz (1961), there are those who suggest that "mental illness" is a myth.

Such sweeping iconoclasm apart, other commentators on the psychiatric scene have called into question the validity of particular diagnostic categories. A seminal paper on classification and the problem of diagnosis is that of McGuire (1973). In his comprehensive review he cites the work of Kreitman et al.(1961) who found that "percentage agreement amongst observers, even when assignment is into fairly broad categories such as organic, functional psychosis, psycho-neurosis, rarely rises above 80%, and when it does it is often possible to detect contamination in that the observers' decisions were not completely independent. When the categories are finer, i.e. diagnosis within the broad groups, agreement fell to around 50% on the average." Considerably earlier, Cameron (1944) had written, "it is important for persons working in the abnormal field to realise that the current official psychiatric classifications are not based upon final and convincing scientific evidence. They are children of practical necessities. Decisions as to the group in which a given behaviour disorder shall fall depend on schemata that actually were adopted, both in (the United States) and Great Britain, by a majority vote of the practicing members of large associations." In the first edition of *The Handbook of Abnormal Psychology* (1958), Eysenck remarked drily that this was an "interesting extension of the democratic process of majority rule into the scientific and medical fields." The more recent, and widely publicised, research of Rosenhan (1973) demonstrates that these concerns about the fallibility of psychiatric diagnosis are still with us. Although Rosenhan was accused of being too extreme in his conclusions about diagnostic carelessness (e.g. Spitzer, 1975; Farber, 1975) he clearly demonstrated how easily mental illness can be feigned.

Equally celebrated, and especially germane, is the paper on Hysteria by Eliot Slater (1965), based on his Shorvon Memorial Lecture, delivered at the National Hospital, London, in 1964. Slater was then Director of the Psychiatric Genetics Research Unit based at the Maudsley Hospital, London. One feels he could be talking about Multiple Personality when he writes "It is generally agreed that none has yet framed a satisfactory definition of 'hysteria'; but it is usually claimed that it can be recognised when met with. However, the ease and reliability with which this is done is differently viewed by different authors." By the end of his carefully argued paper "the gloves are off". Slater concludes that "The only thing that 'hysterical' patients can be shown to have in common is that they are all patients. The malady of the wandering womb began as a myth, and a myth it yet survives. But, like all unwarranted beliefs which still attract credence, it is dangerous. The diagnosis of 'hysteria' is a disguise for ignorance and a fertile source of clinical error. It is in fact not only a delusion but also a snare." (Slater,1965). However, I doubt that, 23 years later, "hysteria" is any the more rarely diagnosed.

Miller (1988) notes that the diagnosis of hysteria conventionally relies on four criteria. Firstly is the presence of symptoms that suggest underlying organic pathology but where no such pathology can be detected, nor is its presence likely. Miller suggests that it is widely accepted that clinicians encounter patients meeting this central and essential criterion from time to time. The remaining criteria, however, are more problematic.

Although the assumption is made that hysterical patients experience secondary gain from their symptoms it is also true that patients with real physical illnesses may experience such gain. They are likely, for example, to receive more care, patience and attention than when they are well.

Classically, hysterical patients are also supposed to exhibit a paradoxical *belle indifférence* to their symptoms but this too is an unreliable indicator. Miller cites Lader and Sartorius (1968) who found that conversion hysterics had elevated anxiety levels which certainly squares with my own clinical experience of such patients.

The focus of Miller's paper, however, is on the fourth criterion, namely the alleged subjective reality of the hysteric's symptomatology. For example, it is assumed that the hysterically blind patient really cannot see, the hysterically paralysed patient really cannot move their limbs. Nor are they consciously aware of the mechanisms that underpin and maintain their symptoms. Such an assumption is essential if we are to distinguish such patients from the consciously simulating malingerer.

Given that we have no access to the contents of each other's consciousness such a criterion clearly raises problems. To put the matter baldly, how can we ever be sure that people are providing accurate and/or truthful subjective reports?

The problem is highlighted by findings such as those of Grosz and Zimmerman (1965) who found that an hysterically blind subject scored less than chance expectation on a visual discrimination task. That is, their subject made fewer correct responses than one would predict from a truly blind subject. This remained the case even when other cues were provided that would have enabled a truly blind subject to identify correctly all the target stimuli. Similarly, Aplin and Kane (1985) found no difference between hysterically deaf patients and subjects asked to simulate on an audiometric test. Such results are consistent with those of Spanos et al. (1985), reported in the previous chapter, where simulators developed secondary personalities like Bianchi, and others with alleged multiple personalities.

Miller refers also to the finding (Silberman et al., 1985) that multiple personality patients show the same degree of interference between personalities from one learning task to another as "normal" controls.

In sum, whatever the clinician's private convictions there seem to be no objective criteria to distinguish between hysteria, or multiple personality, and malingering. Should, then, the distinction be maintained, resting as it does on assumptions about private unconscious and/or dissociative processes? Miller's advice is to remain agnostic as to whether or not the behaviour of the hysteric and the behaviour of the malingerer represent the product of the same, or different, internal processes. This, he says, "opens the way to an emphasis on models of hysteria which do not have to be based on some form of unconscious mental mechanism, and which can lead much more directly to methods of management." As an example, he quotes the model of hysterical symptoms viewed as disturbances in illness behaviour, or inappropriate adoption of the sick-role (e.g. Pilowsky, 1969; Kendell, 1983). Although such positions need careful formulation to avoid tautology they could stimulate research into issues such as "whether those with hysterical symptoms have had greater opportunity than others to experience the benefits of the sick role ... or whether they tend to make different attributions in relation to minor physical symptoms." If such attributional differences were discovered, this could lead to cognitive interventions such as those used in the management of depressed patients.

Despite the attractiveness of Miller's agnosticism, and the undoubted stimulus it should give to researchers, it does present a problem in the context of the present discussion. Choosing to make no distinction between genuine and artificial multiple personalities would inevitably lead to a greatly increased incidence of the diagnosis of this putative disorder. Perhaps just such an implicit agnosticism partly explains the burgeoning number of these patients in the United States.

In contrast to Miller's agnosticism is the more sceptical "atheism" of Mayer-Gross, Slater and Roth (1960) who, in a standard psychiatric text, wrote, "The most superficial form (of hysteria), and one which has attracted much attention from the dramatic form the symptoms take, is seen in the double and multiple personalities, which have been described by Morton prince, McDougall and others. The patient describes herself (*sic*) at different times as being one or another of several different personalities. These different personalities may be endowed with superficially different character traits, and may or may not be aware of each other's existence. Thus a girl who is by turns "Mary" and "Margaret", may be quiet, studious and obedient as Mary, and unaware of Margaret's existence. When she becomes Margaret, however, she may be gay, headstrong and wilful, and refer to Mary in contemptuous terms. It seems that these multiple personalities are always artificial productions, the product of the medical attention that they arouse." These pre-eminent psychiatrists make no further mention of multiple personality in their tome.

In chapter one I referred to fugue states which bear a striking similarity to a major aspect of the multiple personality syndrome, and it will be recalled that it was suggested that Ansel Bourne might have been more appropriately so labelled. However, even this seemingly more conservative diagnosis is not without its critics. In an address given at the National Hospital for Nervous Diseases, London, in 1970, Sir Charles Symonds had this to say:

> I suspect that all so-called hysterical fugues are examples of malingering ... I must have seen half a dozen cases of so-called hysterical fugue in private practice and have adopted the following plan. I have said to the patient "I know from experience that your pretended loss of memory is the result of some intolerable emotional situation. If you will tell me the whole story I promise absolutely to respect your confidence, will give you all the help I can and will say to your doctor and relatives that I have cured you by hypnotism." This approach has never failed, and I have been told some dramatic stories.

One trusts that all psychiatric trainees commit to memory Sir Charles' magic words, although one suspects that multiple personalities are made of rather stronger stuff than the half dozen fugue patients in this post-Chaucerian Knight's Tale.

A paper worthy of more serious consideration has been presented by no lesser authors than Thigpen and Cleckley (1984) themselves. Surprisingly, even these pre-eminent psychiatrists have expressed extreme disquiet about a so-called "epidemic" of multiple personality cases. In a paper that reeks of professional concern they declare that since Eve they have come across only one other case of multiple personality among the tens of thousands of patients they saw in the ensuing 30 years of professional practice. This was not withstanding the hundreds of patients, some who travelled thousands of miles, who strenuously sought to be diagnosed as multiple personality disorders. These protestants went to the lengths of speaking down the telephone in different voices, sending photographs supposed to depict their several selves, and writing letters where the handwriting style changed from paragraph to paragraph. Thigpen and Cleckley tell us that such would-be patients travelled from therapist to therapist until they achieved (sic) the diagnosis and then competed with other patients to have the most personalities. These writers go on to say that "Unfortunately, there also seems to be a competition among some therapists to see who can have the greatest number of multiple personality cases."

They suggest that there are four categories of individual who are responsible for the epidemic of reported cases.

Firstly, there are patients suffering from schizophrenia who are misdiagnosed because the therapist has spent insufficient time with the patient. They remind us that in the case of Eve "it required almost a year of working with her to rule out psychosis." This is a direct challenge to researchers such as Rosenbaum (1980) who believes that vast numbers of multiple personality patients are "missed" by psychiatrists who regard them as schizophrenic. Rosenbaum reviewed the *Index Medicus* from 1903 to 1978 and noted that the diagnosis of multiple personality declined following Bleuler's introduction of the term schizophrenia to replace Kraepilin's "dementia praecox" around 1908. In this way, it is argued that all disorders involving splitting of the personality became subsumed under the one head and the way was paved for the misdiagnosis of multiple personality as schizophrenia. Rosenbaum writes, "The acceptance of the term 'schizophrenia'... was one of the factors related to the decrease in reports of, as well as interest in and recognition of, the multiple personality syndrome. Undoubtedly many other syndromes were (and unfortunately still are) caught in the 'schizophrenic net'." To further support his thesis, Rosenbaum also cites the cases of six individuals with alleged multiple personality whom he believes were wrongly diagnosed as schizophrenic. He goes on to refer to Kirshner's (1973) study of 23 soldiers with dissociative symptoms and amnesia, none of whom were psychotic but four of whom had been previously diagnosed as schizophrenic. Rendon's (1977) research is also quoted where it was reported that Puerto Rican patients with hysterical disorders are likely to be misdiagnosed as schizophrenic. Such references bear a most tenuous relationship to the ostensible main thrust of the paper – namely, the role of the term "schizophrenia" in the decline of diagnoses of multiple personality. Finally, Rosenbaum refers to a handful of textbooks published around 1910 to demonstrate how the term "schizophrenia" usurped "dementia praecox" and became a blanket category for morbid splitting of the personality.

It is a most unconvincing paper based on thin and tortuous argument and I heartily agree with Thigpen and Cleckley (1984) when they say:

> We do not share the view that historically many multiple personality patients were incorrectly diagnosed as schizophrenic, and therefore the incidence of the disorder only appears to have been lower in the past. Schizophrenic patients experiencing hallucinatory or delusional episodes can usually relate the nature of these bizarre ideations and perceptions to the therapist, while the true multiple personality patient experiences total amnesia for the more logical ideations, perceptions, and actions of the alter personalities.

A paper by Bliss, Larson and Nakashima (1983) argues that a principal cause of misdiagnosis are the auditory hallucinations of multiple personality patient deriving from the voices of their latent alter egos. Forty five patients with auditory hallucinations, sequentially identified on admission, constituted the experimental population. Of these, a striking 60% (12 males and 15 females) were diagnosed by Bliss et al. as multiple personalities, and 20 of the 27 had previously been diagnosed as schizophrenic. At first glance this seems to be a more substantive case than that of Rosenbaum until one remarks the following exposition of these researchers' procedure and philosophy:

> The criteria for the diagnosis of multiple personalities proposed in DSM III were not strictly followed, as our experience with over 100 cases of multiple personalities suggests that the present criteria are prematurely rigid and too restrictive. Cases of

multiple personalities vary from blatant examples where personalities are frequently on display, to the subtle cases where personalities can only be identified with certainty via hypnosis. Nevertheless, some of these 'subtle' cases have later revealed as many as 50 personalities. Transformations, the dissociations, are frequently occurring in these patients but the casual observer will see, for example, only tearful, angry, or childish behaviour. Hypnosis will then reveal personalities as the responsible agents, while the patient proves not to be experiencing these altered states because there is a self-hypnotic amnesia or a self-hypnotic dissociation.

Solomon and Solomon (1982) argue that diagnostic confusion can arise because acute schizophrenic patients may simulate multiple personality and, on the other hand, "one of the multiple personality's alterselves may actually be psychotic." One wonders what Solomon and Solomon are implying by the term "psychotic." Given the context they must mean "schizophrenic" which is an a priori impossibility. In what sense could an individual have "selves" that were schizophrenic and selves that were not?

These authors go on to enumerate six diagnostic features which they believe are aids to differential diagnosis between schizophrenia and multiple personality:

1. Schizophrenic patients' auditory hallucinations seem to come from outside whereas the multiple personality experiences them as originating from within.
2. Schizophrenic patients have visual hallucinations whereas multiple personality patients occasionally experience hypnagogic phenomena.
3. Schizophrenics have poor as opposed to intact reality testing (an operational definition of what is meant by such a distinction would seem essential here).
4. Schizophrenic patients have tangential associations accompanied by inappropriate affect whilst the multiple personality patients have circumstantial associations accompanied by appropriate affect (once again, there is clear need for such a distinction to be more explicitly described).
5. Schizophrenic patients establish poor rapport unlike multiple personality patients.
6. Schizophrenia is equally common in males and females compared with the far higher incidence of multiple personality in females.

Those psychiatrists who are confused about the differential diagnosis would also do well to heed the advice of Coons (1984) who writes that "The best way of differentiating schizophrenia from multiple personality is to look for Bleuler's primary symptoms. The schizophrenic has a flat or inappropriate affect, loose or illogical associations, ambivalence, and autism. Although a person with multiple personality may seem indifferent at times, the affect is not flat, and autism, ambivalence, and loose associations do not occur."

Thigpen and Cleckley's second category of patients wrongly called multiple personality are attention-seeking hysterics whose partial dissociations are aggravated by the labelling process. Despite DSM III, Thigpen and Cleckley hold to the view that multiple personality is rooted in hysterical dissociation in the setting of histrionic personalities. It is hard not to sympathise with this traditional association of multiple personality with hysteria remarked upon by Gruenewald (1978) who refers to the nineteenth century coincidence of interests in hysteria, hypnosis and multiple personality. In contrast to Rosenbaum's (1980) speculations about the role of the term "schizophrenia" in this context, she has this to say:

> ... it is not surprising that a great number of cases were found in the early nineteenth century when Mesmerism, the forerunner of hypnosis, was in the ascendancy, and again in the late nineteenth and early twentieth centuries when the French School of Psychiatry espoused hypnosis and hysteria as major interests. It may be no accident that after 1910 significantly fewer cases were reported and that, concurrently, disenchantment with the previously purported powers of hypnosis set in.

Bliss (1980) acknowledges how common were multiple conversion symptoms in a series of 14 multiple personality patients seen over a year, most of whom "qualified for the designation of Briquet's syndrome." Similarly, Coons (1980) states that, "hysterical conversion reactions [in multiple personalities] are almost universal" and cites as examples the numbness, blindness and weakness of Sybil, and the hysterical convulsions of Congdon's (1961) patient, Betty. Solomon and Solomon (1982), whilst suggesting it may be wrong to regard multiple personalities as cases of hysteria, point out that "the patient with multiple personalities typically meets at least some of the DSM III criteria for histrionic personality disorder, such as self-dramatisation, dependency, helplessness, irrational angry outbursts, and tendencies toward manipulative suicidal threats, gestures and attempts."

Thirdly, Thigpen and Cleckley describe a group of individuals who are fundamentally dissatisfied with their self-conception and who dissociate to allow expression to the unacceptable aspects of their personalities. Summarising their sceptical position, and introducing their final category of misclassified individuals, they write, "Before assuming, however, that the patient's 'personalities' or 'ego-fragments' are long-standing, autonomous entities that are fully dissociated from the original personality – and therefore serve separate motives, impulses and feelings – we have found it useful to consider whether there might not be instead a pseudo- or quasi-dissociation that functions to help the patient gain attention, or maintain an acceptable self-image, or accrue financial gain, or even escape responsibility for actions."

This latter reference is specifically to defendants in criminal cases who serendipitously, suddenly emerge as multiple personalities and plead not guilty by reason of insanity. Billy Milligan (referred to in chapter 1) was one such case who was charged with multiple rape. During an interview in prison with psychologist, Dorothy Fuller, the first of nine personalities emerged in response to a direct question about his name. "Billy's asleep," he replied, "I'm David." His largely unchallenged insanity plea was successful and he is currently confined in a psychiatric institution. Thigpen and Cleckley clearly feel that Milligan pulled the wool over the court's eyes; "it is not at all obvious to what extent the court sought to document that a history for, and symptoms indicative of, multiple personality existed prior to this person's arrest ... and [he] was faced with prosecution and punishment for his crimes. We believe from the material at hand that this deliberate manipulation resulted in a gross miscarriage of justice and denigration of psychiatry." More will be said later about multiple personalities in the forensic context which present a peculiarly difficult task for the diagnostician since the motivation for malingering is so obvious.

Even where one is not positing frank malingering, psychopathology is well acquainted with individuals whose presentation is not all that it seems in that it is fuelled by unconscious motivation. In this context one is reminded of the phenomenon of compensation neurosis about which Kennedy (1946), writing in *Compensation Medicine*, had some harsh things to say, "a compensation neurosis is a state of mind born out of fear, kept alive by avarice, stimulated by lawyers and cured by a verdict."

Thigpen and Cleckley conclude their article with this plea, "While there are degrees of dissociation, some of which may be serious enough to require treatment, we urge that the diagnosis of multiple personality disorder be reserved for those very few persons who are truly fragmented in the most extreme manner."

It is hardly surprising that the problem of differential diagnosis has come in for considerable attention. For multiple personality experts regard diagnostic errors as principally responsible for the failure of the vast majority of their colleagues to discover this syndrome in anything like equal numbers, if at all. The issue has been discussed in a number of papers and schizophrenia and histrionic personality disorder are only two of many labels with which it is alleged multiple personality may be confused (e.g. Bliss, 1980; Bliss et al., 1983; Clary et al., 1984; Coons, 1980, 1984; Horevitz and Braun, 1984; Rosenbaum, 1980; Schenk and Bear, 1981; Solomon and Solomon, 1982).

In a study of 40 patients with temporal lobe epilepsy, Schenk and Bear (1981) found that 13 had recurrent dissociative episodes. These took three forms:

1. The patient's attributions to an hallucinated other, often a demon, of their strong affects (exaggerated affective experience is a common characteristic of the interictal syndrome of temporal lobe epilepsy).
2. A tendency to feel they were several different personalities without amnesia.
3. In 3 cases a classic multiple personality syndrome.

In all cases the seizure disorder preceded the dissociative experiences by months or years which led Schenk and Bear to posit a causal mechanism. It is commonly held that a temporal lobe focus leads to new connections between sensory association areas and the limbic system with a resulting heightenening of affect. Schenk and Bear suggest that this leads to dissociation being employed as a defensive mechanism and see partial support for this thesis in the fact that dissociative episodes were always interictal phenomena rather than constituting part of the seizure pattern. They also refer to the findings of Bear and his co-workers (1979, 1980) that ego-alien experiences are often associated with right temporal lobe activation in epileptic patients. This could also lead to dissociative defences which are conventionally associated with overly censorious super-egos.

Mesulam (1981) has also reported dissociative episodes in temporal lobe patients, and fugues have been reported in 78% of such individuals.

Dissociations apart, there are many other similarities between multiple and epileptic personalities such as depressive episodes, overt hostility, altered libido and sexual proclivities (Solomon and Solomon, 1982). The diagnosis of multiple personality should always be preceded by neurological investigations, including a sleep-deprived electroencephalogram with nasopharyngeal leads, to exclude a temporal lobe focus.

An interesting, and frequently vitriolic, flurry of correspondence took place in the Bulletin of the British Psychological Society (January, March, May, and August, 1985) concerning the diagnosis of Breuer's patient, Bertha Pappenheim. Better known as "Anna O", Miss Pappenheim, according to Bliss (1980), "was probably an undetected example of multiple personalities." This likelihood does not seem to have occurred to the correspondents in the BPS Bulletin whose bone of contention was whether or not this famous analysand was suffering from an hysterical neurosis or tuberculous meningitis. The controversy began, on this occasion, when Professor Hans Eysenck took exception to Cooper's review of a new book on Anna O. Ms. Cooper had stated, "that from a severely incapacitated young woman Anna O was enabled to become a vigorous and tireless worker for women's rights. The analysis was impressively successful here." Telling Eysenck that psychoanalysis works has always been a red rag to a bull. Literary nostrils flaring, he replied, "One can only wonder at the level of ignorance displayed by the authors of the book and the reviewer alike. Ellenberger (1972) quoted Jung as saying in 1925 that this famous case, "so much spoken about as an example of brilliant therapeutic was in reality nothing of the kind that ... there was no cure at all in the sense of which it was originally presented." Indeed, as we now know due to the detective work of Hirschmuller (1978), Anna O was not in fact suffering from any kind of psychiatric illness, but from tuberculous meningitis." To the defence of both authors and reviewer came Brett Kahr, the Director of Oxford's Psychoanalytical Forum. His riposte was that tuberculous meningitis is invariably fatal so how did Anna survive until 77, 56 years after her symptoms first presented themselves? The internationally renowned Professor's protestations are dismissed as "pompous and ill-informed diatribes". However, a response from a librarian, Elizabeth Thornton, in the 1985, August Bulletin gave one pause for thought. She argued that it was a fallacy that tuberculous meningitis was "invariably fatal" asserting that 20 cases of recovery were reported in *Brain* (Martin, 1909) when the advent of lumbar puncture had allowed firm diagnosius to be made by microscopic examination of the cerebrospinal fluid for the invasive bacillus. She goes on to say that the course of Anna O's illness was a classic example of the progression of tuberculous meningitis "with initial cough, anorexia and malaise, followed by cranial nerve palsies, and focal signs such as paralyses with contractures, aphasia, cortical visual problems etc." Given that Anna O.'s paralysed limbs were cold and oedamotous and her contractures remained both during sleep and chloral sedation a diagnosis of hysteria does strike one as peculiarly inappropriate (Thornton, 1985).

As well as being confused with an histrionic personality disorder it has been suggested that multiple personality patients may be misdiagnosed as "borderline personalities". Unfortunately, this term is somewhat polymorphous and Horevitz and Braun (1984) have succinctly described the situation as follows:

> Borderline personality has been considered an independent diagnostic entity, a disorder of developmental arrest, a psychostructural disorder defining the boundary between neurosis and psychosis, a set of syndromes with varying genetic bases, a personality disorder related to, but poorly differentiated from, a hysteria/sociopathy cluster, and a mixed set of affective and personality disorders ... The diagnosis of borderline has become a catch-all.

The defining characteristics, according to DSM III, are impulsivity, unstable and intense relationships, inappropriate and intense anger, identity disturbance, emotional instability, intolerance of being alone, physical self-damage, and chronic emptiness or boredom. Although there seems a consensus that differential diagnosis is meaningful (e.g. Solomon and Solomon, 1982; Horevitz and Braun, 1984; Clary et al., 1984), Bliss (1980) has noted that multiple personality patients' responses on a 713 item, self-report questionnaire were very similar to those of borderline patients. Indeed, Solomon and Solomon state that multiple personalities sometimes coexist with borderline personality disorder. Such putative coexistence of two syndromes can only add to the complexity of differential diagnosis and one recalls the remark by Bliss, Larson and Nakashima (1983) that multiple personality may be present alongside schizophrenia.

Horevitz and Braun (1984) cite several writers who have suggested a relationship between multiple and borderline personality (Gruenewald, 1977a,b; Berman, 1977, 1981; Brende and Rinsley, 1981; Clary et al., 1984; Lasky, 1978; Marmer, 1980. However, this must remain a suggestion since the "experimental" populations are woefully small. As the authors note, "For the most part, their work rests on the analysis of one or two cases supplemented by selected case examples from the literature. Clary's discussion of 11 cases seen over a span of 25 years is an exception."

Horevitz and Braun examined the case records of 93 patients and relatives with "confirmed" diagnoses of multiple personality using the Global Assessment Scale of the Schedule for Affective Disorders and Schizophrenia (Spitzer et al., 1979) and the DSM III criteria for Borderline Personality Disorder. These criteria comprise:

1. Intense affects, especially dysphoric angry outbursts and anhedonic and depersonalised states.
2. Impulsivity, especially in drug-seeking, self-destructive behaviour, suicidal gestures, and in areas of sex (promiscuity and frequent paraphilia) and money.
3. Brief psychotic experience.
4. Bizarre response to psychological testing, most notably in unstructured portions

of the WAIS, Bender Visual Motor Gestalt, and in Rorschach tests (for example, F- responses).

5. Good Socialisation, superficially adaptive behaviour masking profound uncertainties regarding identity.

6. Disturbances in close relationships, especially in vacillations between devaluation and idealisation, depressed in the presence of the significant other but responding with histrionic dramatic gestures on threat of abandonment.

7. A predominance of rageful affect in relationships and an inability to tolerate being alone.

The authors say that they were only able to evaluate 33 of the 93 cases, "the remaining 60 had insufficient data for a conclusive evaluation." No more is said about the abandoned 60, and one has to register concern for this kind of presentation of results. The sloppiness of some of the research in the area of multiple personality has already been remarked upon, not unfairly one hopes, and here one reads of the original sample, "with confirmed diagnoses", being excluded for reasons which are quite obscure.

In the event, they found that almost 70% of their sample (23 of 33) also qualified for the diagnosis of borderline personality. In the same symposium, Clary, Burstin and Carpenter (1984) concluded that "multiple personality is a type of narcissistic personality organisation that has much in common with the borderline personality." Clary et al. draw their conclusion from a series of 11 patients who met the 8 criteria already cited in chapter 1, plus one contributed by Clary: "a flatness and lack of vitality in the host personality sometimes taking on an almost somnambulistic appearance." The paper rests on the clinical judgement of the authors who argue for the presence of similarities between the two syndromes within the framework of Object Relations Theory.

Clary et al. note that their findings differ from those of Kluft (1982) who found borderline characteristics in only 22.8% of his 70 patient cohort. The majority are described a "neurotic admixtures" (45%) and "hysterical-depressive" (32%). The proffered explanation for this discrepancy is that Kluft's patients derive from a private psychoanalytic practice and might be assumed to be relatively well functioning given the demands of intensive psychoanalytic psychotherapy. The patients in Clary's sample were poor and referred through public agencies and women's shelters and Kluft (in a personal communication to Clary) says that he sees more borderline personalities in patients referred from such sources. As presented, this is rather anecdotal support for Clary's explanation for the discrepancy between his and Kluft's findings. However, there is nothing new in the idea of high- and low-level pathology (e.g. Kernberg, 1976) amongst neoanalytic theorists. H hysteric, obsessive and depressive disorders are commonly regarded as "higher-level" than, for example, schizoid or borderline personalities. Herzog (1984) suggests that there are high- and low-level multiple personalities and describes the ends of this putative pathological spectrum using two case vignettes, one hysteric and the other schizoid. Kluft (1986) described three "high-functioning" female multiple personality patients, two physicians and a research scientist, with uninterrupted histories of successful professional performance and all experiencing problems in their relationships with men. His stated aim was "not to suggest a new diagnostic category, but to raise the index of suspicion for MPD in apparently stable and successful patients."

It is further argued (Coons, 1984) that multiple personality may not only be confused with schizophrenia, temporal lobe epilepsy and personality disorder (histrionic, antisocial and borderline), but also with other dissociative disorders such as psychogenic amnesia and fugue, as well as depersonalisation disorder and atypical dissociative disorder. However, psychogenic amnesia and fugue usually have clear precipitants, a good prognosis and recurrences are rare. Depersonalisation is not accompanied by amnesia and atypical dissociation is normally experienced by individuals in prisoner or hostage situations who dissociate from the stresses and brutality inflicted by their captors.

Coons (1984) notes too that anxiety, affective and somatoform disorders may also coexist with multiple personality since phobias, mood swings and conversion reactions, such as pseudo-seizures, paralysis and blindness, are all common aspects of the presentation.

Multiple personalities may also exhibit psychosexual disorders such as transsexualism, transvestism, promiscuity and anorgasmia. Bisexuality has been reported in two out of the ten women in Coons' series. One of the women met the Research Diagnostic criteria for alcoholism, and five met the criteria for drug dependence and Coons states that there is a strong association between substance abuse disorders and multiple personality.

Finally, Coons cites an example of factitious dermatological disorder in a woman with a history of a swollen eczematous hand and forearm. It transpired that she had been repeatedly exposing her arm to poison ivy and hitting her left hand.

It is clear that the diagnosis of multiple personality is extraordinarily complex. This is not only because its presentation can be so difficult to distinguish from many other, more familiar, less controversial, syndromes but also because it is alleged that many of these syndromes can coexist with multiple personality. One cannot but sympathise with the likes of Thigpen and Cleckley who believe that it is multiple personality that represents the false-positive diagnosis rather than vice versa; or even with the more extreme position that multiple personality is a chimera. The jaws of scepticism could hardly find a more nourishing trough.

The last paper to receive detailed attention in this chapter was written 25 years ago (Sutcliffe and Jones, 1962) and inevitably suffers from being prepared before the advent of the recent upsurge in alleged cases. Such a dramatic change in diagnostic fashion naturally leads to speculation about the possibility of Type II errors (false positives), even more so when that upsurge is relatively geographically confined. Just such speculation is current in Britain where the North East of England has witnessed a sudden dramatic increase in the diagnosis of child abuse. The paediatricians concerned are involved in legal actions by scores of parents whose children have been taken into care as a result of the doctors's claims. It must be said, of course, that these doctors may well be correct in their diagnoses and simply have greater diagnostic prowess than their counterparts elsewhere. We must await the outcome of the corroborative investigations.

Sutcliffe and Jones identify three phases in the then history of multiple personality. The first is described as hazy beginnings in the early nineteenth century with a few brief reports. The second saw considerable development in the later part of the century centring in France and America and coinciding with great interest in hypnosis and a tendency to explain hypnotic phenomena as multiple personality phenomena. They write, "A self or a personality was a thing-like entity, and there were hidden switches whereby one self could be turned off, and another turned on. Although he did not know how he did it, the hypnotist often manipulated these switches. Psychologists were rather inclined to accept quasi-magical formulations, and this generalised to an acceptance of multiple personality as a like kind of transformation."

The final phase was the acceptance of multiple personality as a diagnostic category and its routine reporting although some doubts were expressed as to its existence in favour of alternative diagnoses.

They explain the peak of interest in the second phase in terms of the prevailing social consciousness which was preoccupied with personal identity and favoured analogies between the human psyche and collectivities of lower organisms which lacked organisation and unity. They further point out that empirical procedures lacked controls, data tended to be anecdotal, findings were inappropriately generalised and theorising was sweeping and ad hoc. The contemporary sceptic might well ask whether we are not still in "phase 3"!

The crudeness of psychiatric diagnosis presented another problem being little more than arbitrary descriptive labelling deriving from the clinicians' predilections. Sutcliffe and Jones write that "with all its faults the current system is at least more systematic than earlier alternatives. There is at least some attempt to limit and define the meaning of terms and the scope of categories. Many cases included as multiple personality in the earlier periods are probably misdiagnosed". They go on to discuss a number of specific cases which they suggest would have been more properly diagnosed as brain damaged, epileptic or schizophrenic. However, even though they subscribe to the view that the diagnosis of multiple personality often represented little more than a diagnostic fad they cautiously concluded that there still remained "a considerable number of cases which might be classified as 'multiple personality' ".

Although multiple personality might be regarded as iatrogenic in the sense that it resulted from the shaping of the patient's behaviour by the therapist they argue that "many of the multiple personality cases exhibited their first alterations without the aid of therapy. Shaping did not therefore fully account for multiple personality." This ignores the issue of whether shaping may have taken place by significant others in these patients' lives, apart from their therapists.

In similar vein, they argue that not all cases arose in hypnotic settings. Thus multiple personality cannot be fully explained as a mere hypnotic artefact. However, they remain impressed by the similarities between hypnotic and multiple personality phenomena. The maintenance of a sceptical view is not, however, solely dependent upon regarding multiple personalities as hypnotic artifacts.

Penultimately, the issue of simulation is raised and here Sutcliffe and Jones present a very abstruse line of thought. They argue that although it could be possible to simulate, consciously or unconsciously, multiple personality behaviours (statements about changed identity, values, tastes, and mood; amnesia, hysterical symptoms and automatisms) these involved "no change in the objective features of the S's 'self'". This cryptic phrase is defined as the individual's "physical being, his actual social role and responsibilities, and his historically verifiable past experience." They argue that conscious simulation normally requires evidence that one is escaping from social pressures, and relies on the collusion of others or the need the absconding criminal might have to assume a new role to escape detection. For reasons that I find completely obscure, Sutcliffe and Jones state that, "the multiple personality patient's assumption of a new identity allows him to escape his own restrictive standards, rather than to conform to the rules or requirements of others. Self-delusion rather than deliberate pretense, would be appropriate to these conditions." This is a most arbitrary piece of the very kind of sweeping and ad hoc theorising which they had earlier condemned. In the ensuing chapter it will be seen that many multiple personality patients explain the emergence of their alter egos precisely because, as children, they were required to conform to the sexual demands of abusing adults. It is mere semantics to argue that the alter ego was born out of conflict with some internal self-concept rather than the objective reality of conflict with a parent bent on incestuous assault.

Finally, these authors raise a crucial issue in a few "thrown away" lines, "the contrast between multiple personality and certain behaviours of normal people was probably too strongly drawn. Normals might be expected to exhibit multiple personality behaviours to some degree." Indeed they might and one asks whether "multiple personality" is ever anything more than the incautious reinforcement by over-eager therapists of a patient's overly dramatised account of the disparate aspects of personality harboured by every human being. Is one witnessing some metaphoric-literal shift whereby the "as-if" is subtly lost along the way? Does the available evidence justify according these patients' alter egos any more existential validity than the reported voices of the hallucinating schizophrenic? My own experience with schizophrenic patients on phenothiazine therapy is that they begin by saying they hear voices "out there", progress to saying that the voices are "inside their heads", and eventually acknowledge that they are "talking to themselves".

This is not to suggest a direct parallel between the schizophrenic who acquires "insight" into his hallucinations as they fade in intensity, and the multiple personality patient whose metaphor for distress is converted into a theatrical display of literal splitting. The two processes are likely to be quite dissimilar, based on the subjective distress of the respective experiences as reported by the patients and the presence or absence of other dissociative phenomena, such as amnesia. I am indebted to Dr Tom Fahy, of the Institute of Psychiatry, University of London, for underlining this distinction (personal correspondence).

CHAPTER 4

How To Bring Up Your Children To Have Multiple Personalities

Discussion of the aetiology of an illness syndrome refers not to a discussion of simple causation but rather to that conglomerate of factors that are seen in some way as precipitating the problem. Such factors can logically be divided into those that are exogenous, such as an external stressor, and endogenous factors, such as an inherited predisposition or a set of attitudes rooted in early socialisation. Or, one may wish to adopt a sceptical position whereby the aetiology is seen as iatrogenic.

A principal reason for questioning the existence of multiple personalities as a discrete clinical entity is their spiralling numbers in the United States contrasted with their virtual absence elsewhere. Those practitioners who are so convinced of the reality of this syndrome belong to a professional subculture with some striking hallmarks as common denominators.

These clinician/researchers generally favour hypnotherapeutic techniques, are psychoanalytic or neoanalytic in orientation, and (deriving from this therapeutic tradition) see their patients intensively, over very long periods of time. Thus it can be argued that the striking similarities between multiple personality phenomena and hypnotic phenomena arise because the former are no more than an artefact of the latter. Similarly, a theoretical preoccupation with the concept of Self (as opposed to, say, Behaviour) and the notion of defensive mechanisms such as repression, dissociation and splitting, might suggest that multiple personality is more in the eye of the psychoanalytically inclined therapist than in the psyche of the analysand. Victor (1975) responding to Barbara's (1974) review of "Sybil", writes, "I would suggest that the likelihood of a diagnosis of multiple personality ... being made is positively correlated with the romantic and fanciful tendencies of the diagnostician."

The intensity and duration of the therapy could only aggravate such a state of affairs. Indeed, the length of therapy has been used by such therapists as an explanation as to why it is only they who uncover these cases. It has been argued that multiple personalities have spent their lives hiding from others (including the "host personality") their alter egos. Therefore, such alter egos would be expected to emerge only after lengthy treatment when, inter alia, the patient feels sufficiently safe in the therapeutic relationship to fully disclose themselves. A normal corollary is that the diagnosis of multiple personality is only possible within the confines of just such a therapeutic alliance. This is yet another idiosyncracy of the field multiple personality since it is common practice to act solely as diagnostician, even feeling that one's detachment from a therapeutic involvement allows for greater objectivity. Clinical psychologists frequently operate in just such a diagnostic capacity. The sceptic's natural cynicism is only nurtured by being told that the recognition of this disorder is exclusive to acolytes who are actively involved in the treatment of such cases. Such a stricture smacks of ideology rather than science.

There is a general consensus in the literature that alternate personalities first emerge during childhood (Greaves, 1980; Bliss, 1980; Boor, 1982). Putnam et al. (1986), reviewing 100 cases, reported that "in 28 patients, no age was recorded; of the remaining 72, 89% retrospectively reported that the first appearance of an alternate personality occurred before age 12 years. The mean age at first appearance was 5.98 years (range, 1–32, median = 4 years)." Greaves (1980) informs us that, in a personal communication, Allison has suggested that there may be "two major forms" of multiple personality depending on whether the alternates first emerged during the period 0–8, or 8–16 years. In the former case the likelihood would be a large number of personalities since the splitting is seen as coinciding with a stage when the ego is relatively unformed.

Splitting during the latter period would produce relatively few personalities. The problem with such data is that they are based on the necessarily retrospective accounts of the patients and it is not necessary to elaborate on the pitfalls inherent in data so exposed to the vicissitudes of human memory.

A further problem resides in Allison's hypothesis which requires that one counts the number of personalities in a given patient. This is no straightforward matter for a number of reasons. Firstly, it has already been seen that there exist no objective criteria to help one decide whether a given set of behaviours constitute a "personality". Authors have incorporated into their definitions such epithets as "well developed", "integrated", "complex", "distinct", apparently oblivious to the fact that these terms are all but meaningless. And into the midst of this terminological bedlam came Coons (1984) to draw a distinction between "personality" and "personality fragment." It really is painfully reminiscent of ancient theologians debating how many angels could sit on a pin-head. However, Putnam et al.(1986) soberly report that they asked clinicians to complete a questionnaire asking them to write down the number of "distinct and separate" (*sic*) personalities in their patients of which they were aware. They go on to inform us that numbers "ranged between 1 and 60; five therapists reported being unable to count the number of alternates in their patients. The mean number of personalities was 13.3, the median was 9, and the mode was 3." One has to sympathise with the band of five who could not come up with a number. Perhaps they, too, felt that the final figures, albeit dignified with some simple descriptive statistical tags, would not mean too much.

The second problem inherent in "counting" personalities is knowing just when to stop. Eve, for example, is famous for her "three faces" but recounted a further 19 which emerged after her discharge from therapy. Bliss (1986) acknowledged this "growth potential" when he wrote of a patient that she had "at last count almost fifty (personalities)." The implication is also clear that the number of personalities "discovered" is partly a function of both the credulity and therapeutic prowess of the clinician concerned. One fears that counting alter egos, as with angels, is no task for the uninitiated.

It has been frequently reported that these early personalities began as imaginary playmates who then metamorphosed into "selves" with independent existences beyond the control of their hosts. A species of guests, one might say, who outstay their welcome. However, the "presence" of such imaginary companions cannot be used as a prognosticator since so many children indulge in such fantasies. Pines (1978), writing in *Psychology Today*, cites a study where 65% of a sample of a normal population of nursery school and day-care centre children, aged between 2 and 10 years, who had just such "invisible playmates" (*sic*). However, consistent with the reported preponderance of female multiple personality patients, Jersild et al. (1933) found that girls were more likely to have such companions, and they also tended to have a higher IQ than those who did not.

Given that any aetiological account will necessarily deal with the interaction between both exogenous and endogenous factors one might ask what life events characterise those children whose personalities disintegrate. Boor (1982) answers as follows: "Arduous standards of conduct required by severely restrictive environments, coupled with severe family discord, parental psychopathology, physical abuse, sexual trauma, and parental absence or rejection...." It is argued that such circumstances lead to endogenous precipitants, namely guilt, ambivalence and problems in expressing anger or sex. Greaves (1980), duly acknowledged by Boor, had already written "the two principal contributory factors to multiple personality, recurringly mentioned by observers, are a psychic and environmental atmosphere of extreme ambivalence and the experience of major psychic/or physical trauma." Boor also speculates that the sex bias reflects the inability of females in society to act out their conflicts owing to repressive socialisation, as well as reflecting the greater dissonance in role demands that women experience. The problem inherent in such sociological speculation is that it is extraordinarily difficult to operationalise and translate into scientific investigation. For the moment it might best be regarded as a journalistic aside.

Child abuse has received considerable attention in the multiple personality literature and there are certainly some horrendous tales in the histories of these patients. Kluft, addressing the American Psychiatric Association in 1979, put it baldly when he said, "I see multiple personality as a syndrome which follows child abuse. Most multiples, as children, have been physically brutalised, psychologically assaulted, sexually violated, and affectively overwhelmed. A small number may have only experienced one of these forms of personal desecration." Putnam et al. (1986) state, "a history of significant childhood trauma, generally in the form of child abuse, was noted in the majority of MPD patients reported in our study." The most commonly reported trauma was sexual abuse (83%), typically incest (68%). Also reported was repeated physical abuse (75%), both sexual and physical abuse (68%). As if this were not enough a striking 45% had witnessed, as children, the "violent death, usually of a parent or sibling."

Allison (1974), in a paper whose title inspired the present chapter head ("A Guide To Parents: How To Raise your Daughter To Have Multiple Personalities"), enumerates seven "rules":

1. Don't want the child in the first place.
2. Create and strengthen polarity between mother and father.
3. Make sure one parent, especially the favoured one, disappears before the child is 6 years old.
4. Encourage sibling rivalry, or at least don't recognise it or help your daughter deal with it.
5. Be ashamed of your family tree.
6. See to it that her first sexual experience is traumatic and that she can't tell you about it.
7. Make sure her home life as an adolescent is so miserable she wants to get married to get away. Then allow her to marry a sexual deviate who can carry on in your tradition.

In an aetiological study of eight multiple personality patients, Stern (1984) found that all were the victims of child abuse. All had been physically abused, amounting to torture in five cases. Six had been sexually abused, five by family members. Saltman and Solomon (1982) also present a series of patients exhibiting multiple personalities where all six had suffered violent incest in family settings characterised by unstable and impoverished interpersonal relationships and family role confusion. They remind us of Sybil who suffered the ambivalent attitudes of a father who was "so sexually prudish that he would not allow her to sit on his lap, yet she was permitted to witness her parents engage in sexual intercourse" (Saltman and Solomon, 1982). They further cite the finding of Rosenbaum and Weaver (1980) that the majority of the 33 papers on multiple personality published between 1934 and 1978 reported incest and other sexual trauma in the childhood of the victims.

Rene, whose case history forms the core of Confer and Ables' (1984) book, reported being raped by her alcoholic father when she was 11, as well as being pressed to cunnilingus with her mother and witnessing her father having sexual relations with a live-in babysitter.

Bliss (1986, p.136) states that "brutal treatment by parents, sexual molestation, and other disasters are commonly reported and (although) it has not been possible to establish the veracity of these experiences in all patients ... in thirteen subjects collateral evidence was available from parents, siblings, and other sources." However, not all multiple personality patients have suffered such assaults, Eve being a famous case in point. There is a crying need for longitudinal research which would follow up the life careers of the dramatically increasing number of victims of child abuse. Only in this way could one be confident about making predictions such as that of Wilbur (1984) when she asserts, "when child abuse is controlled, the number of multiple personality disorder patients will decline."

Arising from this gamut of sexual trauma and disturbed family dynamics it is not surprising that writers have postulated that the child victims grow into adults with extreme difficulties in the expression of anger and sex. Thus one could predict that alter egos will normally have amongst their number those that express these repressed conflicts. Alternates are commonly sexually provocative, even promiscuous, as well as hostile and sometimes physically violent (obviously presenting special challenges in the treatment situation).

Putnam et al. (1986) record that, "outwardly directed violence is also frequently reported in this disorder. Alternate personalities who were described as assaultive or destructive were found in 70% of cases. Homicidal behaviour attributed to a specific alternate personality was reported in 29% of cases, and actual homicides were allegedly committed by six patients. Twenty per cent of the patients were said to have been involved in a sexual assault on another individual."

One thinks of Jonah (Brandsma and Ludwig, 1974), a patient with four personalities. One, "King Young", was described as "a smooth talking hedonist who is very heterosexually orientated." A second, "Usoffa Abdulla", emerged when Jonah was physically attacked as a boy and "his duty is to protect Jonah. He is cold, belligerent, sullen and scary to interview. He is the 'warrior' who handles angry feelings by decisive, aggressive action." Perhaps the most dramatic case of such sexual and aggressive "acting out" was Kenneth Bianchi, whose murderous exploits have already been discussed in Chapter 2.

Winer (1978) documents the case of Nancy whose multiple personalities she construed as arising directly from Nancy's inability to express her anger. Nancy certainly had a traumatic history. Her parents married and divorced four times and the marriages were characterised by violent episodes. Her mother attacked Nancy's father and grandfather with knives, and once wrestled over a shotgun with Nancy's father resulting in the gun blowing a hole in the ceiling. Her mother seduced both the first boyfriend, and the first husband of her daughter, and, in a drunken rage, even tried to kill Nancy and her two children with a knife. Rather than retaliate, Nancy would run away from such situations and react with hurt and disappointment rather than anger. Winer's hypnotherapy involved putting Nancy "in touch" with her alternate, Kitty, who harboured all Nancy's repressed hostility towards her mother. Winer concluded that Nancy had been unable to express her own violent feelings because, "Although it is common for children to grow angry at their mothers, in few cases would the anger result in annihilation. When Nancy grew up, she saw as her only model of anger the murderous rage of her mother, completely out of control, which resulted in the destruction of the family. Such a violent, unpredictable mother might retaliate with either abandonment or murder at the first sight of anger in her daughter. Either of these reactions would result in annihilation for the child. So the child, when she could not longer hide the anger from herself, really split to survive."

Boor's (1982) review cites a number of other case reports where conflict in the expression of anger and/or sex are regarded as significant in the aetiology of multiple personalities (Bliss, 1980; Boor, 1981; Brende and Rinsley, 1981; Danesino, Daniels and McLaughlin, 1979; Kjervik, 1979; Lasky, 1978; Pohl, 1977; Price and Hess, 1979; Smith and Sager, 1971). For the most part, these reports are extremely brief, and the question arises of selectivity in reporting.

Given that all child victims of abuse and variants of family psychopathology, even those who cannot express their anger, do not develop multiple personalities, one must ask what is the contribution of other, perhaps endogenous factors?

The distinction between endogenous (biological and psychological) and exogenous factors is not always clear cut. A set of pathological external circumstances could be seen as producing psychological attitudes which would inhibit normal personality development and/or social relationships. An illustration would be the "double-bind" hypothesis of Bateson whereby a family atmosphere of ambivalence and contradictory communications is posited as leading to mistrust in the child; mistrust not only of further communications from others but also of one's own ability to select appropriate coping strategies from one's response repertoire. Laing took this further and argued that an extreme reaction to such a bind was schizophrenic breakdown.

Also, the distinction between aetiological discussion and theoretical explanation can become blurred. Thus a full account of internal and external precipitants together with an explicit description of how these produce the defining signs and symptoms of a disorder amounts to a theory of that disorder.

It is easier to keep aetiology and theory distinct when one is dealing with accounts of external events. Thus one can say that a normal precursor of multiple personality is child abuse, without venturing into discussion of causal links. However, statements about internal events, of necessity, trespass into the realm of theoretical speculation. Unless one is dealing with relatively simple biological reactions to external agents, one must have recourse to a language of "theoretical constructs" and "intervening variables" (MacCorquodale and Meehl, 1948) and what are these but convenient, temporary fictions? Such concepts are different not only because of the private worlds they inhabit, their intrinsic mentalism ("cognitive dissonance" will suffice as an example), but more importantly, because they derive their meaning from their position in some theoretical system. Behaviourist and psychoanalyst can agree that violent incest occurs with uncommon frequency in the history of multiple personality patients. Violent incest needs no coy enclosure in quotation marks. However, it is a different question if one wants to posit endogenous aetiological factors such as "psychic readiness", "proneness to splitting" or "hypnotisability". Trade in such conceptual currency requires both knowledge of their theoretical contexts, as well as an ideological commitment.

This brief excursion into the philosophy of science is to explain why treatment of the endogenous triad – psychic readiness, proneness to splitting and hypnotisability – will inevitably make some early incursions into the more focused discussion of theories of multiple personality to which a later chapter is devoted.

"Psychic readiness" is Greaves' (1980) term and derives explicitly from the framework of ego-psychology. He argues that infants begin by construing the world from a hedonistic, undifferentiated point of view when they are absorbed in their own "autarchic" fantasies, akin to Freud's "primary process" thinking. The ego is born out of conflict with an external reality which has a habit of frustrating immediate gratification and thereby imposes an awareness of its presence on the maturing infant. There then follows a stage when these external "objects", with their "good" and "bad" aspects, are incorporated, or internalised. In this way, the ego develops its own sense of separateness and identity, and autarchic functioning is replaced by relational functioning. However, (quoting Greaves) "What seems to happen in the borderline states is that the process of object relations formation, essential to the development of both a sense of self and a mature ego, becomes extremely disrupted." This disruption arises because parental neglect leads to regression to a narcissistic stage of development ("if they, out there, can't satisfy my needs, I'll rely on my own resources"). Also, such parents will provide inadequate models for introjection, and, to the extent that they are internalised, an ego will be formed replete with "bad" objects. Such an ego will be "unstable ... laden with chronic anxiety, (tending) to decompensate under stress, and ... characterised by poor interpersonal bonding and major interpersonal anxiety over issues of intimacy and trust" (Greaves, 1980).

Things could be even worse, Greaves suggests, if the transitional infant were exposed not just to painful but to "high intensity, emotionally provocative, and contradictory stimuli." Along with Freud, he posits that this would lead to the formation of an ego which was fragmented, with its different identifications being cut off from each other, "the different identifications (seizing) hold of consciousness in turn" (Freud, in *The Ego and the Superego*, 1923). The ego is now "psychically ready" for splitting as a defensive manoeuvre. However, Greaves believes that it is important to distinguish the splitting seen in borderline, from that in multiple, personalities. The former have an organisation which is diffuse, non-integrated, fractured and unstable, but lack the separateness and encapsulation seen in the alter egos of the multiple personality victim. Greaves explanation is such a delightful piece of Lewis Carollian gobbledygook that I quote it in full. He says:

> The difference appears to be this. ... In borderline personality, there is both a poverty of object relations and a highly diffuse, fragmented ego, lacking in a stable central core, arising out of the failure to integrate painful and chaotic introjects. However, in multiple personality something different happens, namely, that in the process of cathecting disorganised percepts to pools of polarised affect, a form of personality organisation results which is quite unlike other borderline states.

If one is not yet clear about this distinction, Greaves helps further: "In other words, alter selves, though woefully incomplete as personality systems, may nevertheless represent a level of ego organisation which is higher than that of borderline personality." Leaving aside this allusion to "woefully incomplete personality systems" (whatever happened to Taylor and Martin's "complex and integrated [personalities] each with its own unique behaviour patterns and social relationships"?), it would be generous to describe Greaves' account as an "explanation." It is no more than the crudest adhockery which rather than address itself to characteristic differences in the "splitting" per se, simply tells us that the resulting personality organisation is "quite unlike" that seen in borderline states. If one asks, "In what way 'unlike'?", the answer is that the level of organisation in multiples is "higher" than that seen in borderlines.

This kind of circular description, especially in such abstruse language, cannot count as any sort of scientific explanation, which is not to dismiss Object Relations Theory (ORT) and attendant notions such as "splitting".

The association between multiple personality and hypnosis dates back to the nineteenth century French school of psychiatry and Janet (1889) who conceived of multiple personality as an hysterical disorder involving spontaneous self-hypnosis. Bliss (e.g. 1980, 1986) is the leading contemporary proponent of this view that multiple personality is "the subject's unrecognised abuse of self-hypnosis." Appropriately, Greaves (1980) suggested that "it would be useful to establish whether persons with multiple personality are particularly susceptible to hypnosis as is widely believed", in other words, whether "hypnotisability" could be invoked as an endogenous aetiological factor. Apart from a priori argument based on certain similarities between hypnotic and multiple personality phenomena, Bliss and Jeppsen (1985) believe they have empirical evidence for such a relationship. Six inpatients meeting the DSM III criteria for multiple personality completed the Stanford Hypnotic Susceptibility Scale (Form C) (Weitzenhoffer and Hilgard, 1962) and had a mean score of 10.2 ± 0.65. This is a high score, occurring in less than 10% of the normal population. However, the authors acknowledge that the sample is extremely small. One also has misgivings when the DSM III criteria alone are used since they do not include amnesia. Amnesia is a sine qua non for diagnosis if one is arguing for a qualitative difference between the phenomenology of multiple personality patients and everyday awareness that one's personality is multi-faceted. Jeppsen also "clinically judged" nine outpatients (also diagnosed as multiple personalities using DSM III criteria) to be "excellent hypnotic subjects". The authors go on to say, "The reliability of his clinical judgement was studied on eight other patients who he identified as excellent hypnotic subjects. They scored 9.9 ± 0.55, on the (Stanford) test, a very high score that confirmed the reliability of his clinical judgement." The authors mean "validity" rather than reliability, and it is a pity that more direct evidence, based on a larger sample of subjects, who all evidenced amnesia, is not available. In fairness to Bliss and Jeppsen, they are aware of some methodological defects and state, "This survey ... was restricted to inpatients on two university acute psychiatric wards and to outpatients referred to a psychiatrist who uses hypnosis and has treated many patients with multiple personality. Whether the results are representative of the general population of patients treated on acute units and as outpatients by psychiatrists can only be determined by further studies."

At this stage one must caution that there are obvious dangers in explaining one mysterious and elusive phenomenon, namely multiple personality, in terms of an equally mysterious and elusive phenomenon, that of hypnosis. Neurological evidence that hypnosis is a "state" (e.g. White, 1941) rather than role playing (e.g. Sarbin and Andersen, 1967) is wanting and it could be argued that no critical experiment could be devised to distinguish between these two formulations. Evidence which relies on physiological correlates such as altered electroencephalograms is dogged by the problem of the primogeniture of chicken and egg. A more radical problem is that of scientific ideology. Perhaps the only acid test of whether or not a subject is "really" hypnotised as opposed to role playing, or even simulating, is to ask them to describe their subjective experience. Presumably, adopting a social role, or "pretending" somehow "feels different" from being in a passive, altered state of consciousness, when, for example, normally voluntary motor movements seem to occur outside conscious control. Such introspective data are neither sought nor given much credence by behaviourists. Thus rather than reformulate multiple personality in terms of hypnosis one would expect researchers like Spanos et al.(1986) to subsume both of these phenomena under a head such as role playing which is more consistent with the position of a social learning theorist.

Gruenewald (1984), citing Bliss's (1980) view that multiple personality is "the subject's unrecognised abuse of self-hypnosis", notes that acceptance of such a position is dependant on one's operational definition of hypnosis. In her thoughtful paper comparing hypnosis with multiple personality, she says that although "Hypnosis-like phenomena do appear spontaneously and may be inadvertently utilised in various ways ... such phenomena are deemed analogous to but not identical with hetero- and self-hypnosis."

More will be said in the ensuing theoretical discussion about the respective positions vis à vis hypnosis and multiple personality of Bliss, Spanos, Gruenewald, and Braun (1984) who argued tendentiously that "there is no evidence that hypnosis can produce multiple personalities."

Let us allow Stern (1984) the closing, summary remarks on the knotty problem of aetiology. Paraphrasing from his paper, there are four categories of explanation of multiple personality:

1. Supernatural, such as spirit possessions and reincarnation, which are still current in certain cultures and religious groups.
2. Physiological, such as interrupted blood supply to certain cerebral lobes or epilepsy, where he finds the evidence sparse and inconclusive.
3. Sociological, under which head he subsumes role playing theories.
4. Psychological.

Under the last heading the theories abound and he enumerates such notions as "psychologic feebleness", "ego weakness", "lowered general energy", "personification of the superego", "various identifications of the ego", "repression", "primitive wish-fulfilment", "regression", "early conflicting parental introjects", and the personification of sexual impulses. However, he rightly objects that all of these are based upon the clinician investigator's preconceived theoretical positions and most of the concepts preclude rigorous examination.

Stern (1984) offers 15 hypotheses which he combines into what he calls a paradigmatic description of the aetiology of multiple personality disorder:

1. Child abuse or neglect.
2. A background that includes rigid religious or mystical beliefs.
3. Contradictory communications from significant others during childhood.
4. Above-average intelligence in subjects.
5. Severe pathology exhibited in at least one caretaker.
6. The first split occurring in childhood.
7. Identity confusion in the subject in childhood.
8. High stress in social interactions at the time each split occurred.
9. Extreme anxiety and confusion in subjects.
10. Only a few hours or days between a split and its crystallisation as a complete entity.
11. Personalitities' names derive from identifications with others and childhood fantasy figures.
12. Each personality has a function or purpose to carry out.
13. Many personalities try to hide their identities from other people.
14. Personalities hide their existence from the host who denies their presence.
15. Many multiple personality subjects believe in parapsychologic experiences and in spirits. Some claim past lives and spirit possessions as the origin of their alternate personalities.

In a study of just eight subjects, Stern found that all hypotheses, save 13 and 14, stood up. However, he believes that alternate personalities tended to "come out" more readily than supposed, although they might not reveal they had a different name from the host. Stern concludes that what actually happens is that the host personality denies the existence of alternates rather than the latter deliberating hiding from view. Such speculation is surely no less difficult to examine rigorously than the other psychological notions about which Stern was so sceptical?

It would be interesting to explore further the relationship with paranormal beliefs and reported experiences such as déjà vu, precognition and out-of-the-body experiences. It is this author's clinical experience that such beliefs are also common in hysterical subjects but for the present such hunches must await less anecdotal support.

It seems clear that multiple personality patients typically report a history of childhood trauma and abuse, the latter normally involving sexual assault. Indulgence in imaginary playmates is too common to serve as a distinguishing characteristic. It is also likely, if multiple personality rally is a discrete clinical entity, that endogenous factors remain to be elicited and identified. There have been a limited number of objective studies of multiple personality patients, together with speculation about the physical underpinnings of this disorder and these are the focus of the next chapter.

CHAPTER 5

Objective Approaches to Multiple Personality

So far the focus has been on clinical and semantic issues. It has been suggested that the use of differing diagnostic criteria makes it difficult to know if one is comparing like with like when looking at the various case studies. There is also the problem that at least some of the patients diagnosed as multiple personalities may be suffering from some other illness, for example, fugue, schizophrenia, borderline personality disorder, or an organic syndrome.

The problem is not simply whether or not multiple personality "exists". Clearly, there are a large number of individuals who describe their psyches as being fractured into many disparate selves, and as being amnesic for much of their behaviour. The problem is more one of deciding what alternative classifications might be employed to subsume such clinical presentations. There is considerable consensus that the aetiology of multiple personality involves traumatic childhood experiences in a context of ambivalent and conflictful family relationships where significant others are evidencing extreme psychopathology. However, caution is necessary when evaluating data that rely so heavily on retrospective accounts. In addition, one knows that other psychiatric syndromes can result from such tragic histories, that not all individuals with such backgrounds become psychiatrically ill, and that not all multiple personality patients have endured such trauma. Indeed, one has every sympathy with the clinical investigators trying to arrive at an unequivocal diagnosis. Their difficulties can only be confounded by the knowledge that their patients, even if not simulating, may be producing symptoms that are artefacts of the strenuous and exhausting therapeutic endeavours used to help them. It is only fair to reiterate that many of the criticisms and caveats rehearsed in earlier chapters have come from those who are none the less convinced of the clinical utility of "multiple personality" as a discrete diagnosis.

Perhaps the most notable critics are Thigpen and Cleckley themselves who made no bones about saying that multiple personality has been grossly overdiagnosed in the last three decades.

However, there have been attempts to place multiple personality on somewhat surer ground. These have taken the form of experimental investigations and the search for possible physiological and psychological test correlates of this disorder and it is to this research that the present chapter is directed.

An early study was that of Condon, Ogston and Pacoe (1969) who analysed, frame by frame, a 30 minute film of Eve, made by Thigpen and Cleckley. The film was viewed in the search for possible facial regularities as well as other transformations of expressive behaviour. During the film, Eve White, Eve Black, and Janes I and II all presented themselves. (Condon et al. note that Jane displayed two aspects, hence their subdivision into "I and II"). What the authors observed in all personalities was a transient microstrabismus (the deviation of one eye from the axis of the other). One eye might move to the left whilst the other remained still. Or both eyes might diverge simultaneously to the left and right. Finally, while both eyes are moving in the same direction one eye might move markedly faster than the other.

During the first 4½ minutes of film no explicit identification of personalities occurred and there were only three instances of strabismus. However, there were 73 instances of strabismus during the remaining 25½ minutes distributed as shown in Table 5.1.

Qualitatively, the authors noted that for Eve White, the left eye tended to move divergently while the right eye remained still. Eve Black revealed a tendency to right-eye movements and Jane I's eye tended to move right for one frame and then back left again on the next.

Condon et al. recall that Anna O. evidenced some visual disturbance at the onset of her illness, a convergent squint with diplopia, and deviation of both eyes to the right when reaching for something so that her hand always went to the left of the object. They further recall, in the case of Miss Beauchamp, that "Sally" would concentrate on peripheral vision whilst Miss Beauchamp would focus on central vision. Given that

TABLE 1

Distribution of Strabismus Between Personalities (from Condon, Ogston and Pacoe, 1969)

Personality	Frequency of Strabismus	Time each personality appears in film
Eve White	11	7 min.
Eve Black	56	9 min.
Jane I	6	4 min.
Jane II	0	2½ min.
Total	73	

disturbances of oculomotor parallelism have also been noted in some schizophrenic patients, and that this form of strabismus has not been observed in normals, these tentative findings warrant further investigation. The authors conclude, "Such clinical observations suggest the possibility of a more than purely semantic relationship between the dissociation of a personality and the dissociation of normal oculomotor parallelism."

It is well established that visual disturbances can be associated with headaches, as migraine victims know to their cost, and reports of headache are common in the accounts of multiple personality patients. Bliss (1980), in his study of 14 multiple personality patients, found that 91% of patients complained of severe headaches as compared with 23% of control subjects. In their cohort of 100 such patients, Putnam et al. (1986) record that headaches predominated among medical symptoms, being noted in 65% of cases. Eve was originally referred because of "severe and blinding headaches" and Sybil had headaches "so bad that following such an attack [she] had to go to sleep for several hours [as if] drugged" (Schreiber, 1973). Faith (Larmore et al., 1977) complained of "severe headache beginning in the left temporal area which would settle at the top of her head like a vice." Jonah (Ludwig et al., 1972), when first admitted, complained chiefly of "severe headaches for variable periods of time" and, like Faith, these would be followed by amnesia. Rene, described by Confer and Ables (1983), also suffered from headaches which were prodromal to dissociation. In the forensic context, Forsyth (1939) documents the case of a "middle-aged embezzler" suffering from dual personality who experienced "a series of bad headaches" accompanied by depression and withdrawal. It would be tedious to say more about other researches (e.g. Gruenewald, 1971; Wagner and Heise, 1974; Allison, 1978) which have found this association between multiple personality and severe headaches which is, at least, suggestive of an organic component in this syndrome.

Reports of EEG studies on multiple personalities are few and their findings equivocal. Thigpen and Cleckley (1954) found that two of Eve's three personalities provoked normal EEGs, and the third was borderline-normal although distinguishable. However, as Coons et al. (1982) point out, their recording session was only 33 minutes and provided only short samples of each personality. The objective study of Faith by Larmore et al. (1977) produced inconclusive findings relating to alpha activity recorded with eyes open and closed. They also found little difference in contingent negative variation records between Faith's four personalities. Ludwig et al. (1972), whose patient also had four personalities, report that alpha blocking with eye opening figured consistently in the records of "Jonah" and "Sammy" but not in those of "King Young" and "Usoffa Abdullah." They concluded "That the fact that these (quantitative data) show patterns in different states not readily explainable on differences in alertness suggests real physiologic differences." In Chapter 8 Spanos et al. (1985) call this conclusion into question.

In contrast, Coons et al. (1982) found no basic EEG changes as the different personalities were elicited in their two subjects. In fact, more differences were evident between the simulated personalities of a control subject. Thus they felt that the differences were attributable to changes in emotional state, involving degree of concentration and muscle relaxation, and it was not "as if each personality is a different individual with a different brain." A number of EEG studies on multiple personalities are in progress in the United States, at NIMH, and one awaits their outcome with interest.

Given that some kind of "splitting" is a hallmark of multiple personality it was predictable that some authors would seek to operationalise such a polymorphous concept. There has been speculation that the mechanism may be a functional impairment within the corpus callosum which interferes with communication between the cerebral hemispheres. Accordingly, Brende (1984) has postulated that different personalities involve different hemispheres and may be lateralised in the following hypothetical way:

1. A protective personality whose "role" would be to defend against environmental threat and awareness of disturbing imagery, emotions, and recollections of post-traumatic events would probably be associated with the cognitive, unemotional, and defensive functions of the left hemisphere.

2. A victim personality who experiences repetitive re-enactments of disturbing post-traumatic events would probably be associated with the right hemisphere's non-cognitive functioning and emotionally charged imagery of traumatic events.

3. "Splitting" is a mental mechanism that maintains separation between the defensive qualities of a parental "protective" personality "housed" within the left hemisphere and a child-like victim personality "housed" within the right hemisphere.

4. Dissociation (or switching) is a physiologically based mechanism, resulting from functional disruption of neurotransmitter communication between each of the hemispheres, thus resulting in selective functioning of personalities linked to either hemisphere in response to specific control or expressive needs of the whole organism.

Brende then refers to the defensive mechanisms, "over-control" and "under-control" (Horowitz and Becker,1972), for example, amnesia or denial contrasted with intrusive, disturbing images. Gellhorn and Kiely (1972) has speculated that the physiological basis of these mechanisms may lie in the inhibition/excitation balance, the former involving cholinergic, and the latter catecholaminergic transmitters. Brende, therefore, hypothesises that at least one personality will be dedicated to over-control, serving a protective, defensive role, and its presence will be activated by cholinergic transmitters. This personality would be "housed" in the left hemisphere. At least one other personality, activated by catecholamines, would exist in a state of under-control, re-enacting traumatic experiences, and would be "housed" in the right hemisphere.

To test these hypotheses, Brende made bilateral electrodermal response (EDR) measurements in a single patient with three personalities. He chose EDR measurement because "The presence of specific emotional and behavioral symptoms in association with EDR lateralisation suggests the likelihood of a relationship between cerebral and EDR lateralisation", (Brende, 1984). From Lacroix and Comper's (1979) study, it seems that stimulus- evoked electrodermal assymetry is under the control of the contra-lateral hemisphere so that decreased left EDRs would follow right-hemisphere activation.

It was found that the emergence of the unemotional, protective personality was, indeed, associated with such a decrease in left-sided EDRs. The emergence of the "victim personality" was associated with increases in left-sided EDRs. Brende concludes "As these two personalities remained clearly differentiated from each other, the lack of integration of cognitive and emotional "roles" continued to promote frequent dissociations, revealed in this study to be not only between personalities, but almost certainly between cerebral hemispheres as well." Such a conclusion, drawn from an uncontrolled single-case study, and based on very speculative theorising, must remain tentative. One awaits others who will follow Brende's imaginative lead.

Equally tentative must be the finding of Mathew et al. (1985), who measured regional cerebral blood flow in a patient with two alternate personalities (see Meyer, 1978, for a technical description of the methodology, known as X133 Yenon inhalation). The premorbid personality was designated "A" and the two alternates, "B" and "C." Following blood-flow measurement for personality "A" the patient was hypnotised and personality change to "B" induced using hypnosis. She was then instructed to come out of her "trance" so that measurement could be taken when not under hypnosis. For reasons which the authors do not explain, "cerebral blood-flow measurements could not be carried out for personality 'C' ." The personalities are reported as "fusing" after 3 weeks of in-patient treatment and "at the time of discharge the final personality, personality 'D', was that of a relatively stable woman who had come to terms with her unpleasant childhood memories ... of severe verbal, physical and sexual abuse." Mathew et al. state that blood-flow values are highly reliable for individuals and readings from personalities "A" and "D", together with those from three control subjects, illustrated this. "However, the values of personalities 'A' and 'B' showed more marked differences even though the measurements were made back-to-back and with the same (30 minute) time interval as that used in the control runs." These authors found that personality change was associated with increased temporal lobe blood flow in the right hemisphere. They believe that, since they had carefully excluded temporal lobe epilepsy, this increase more likely reflected functional overactivity.

In a well-designed study of 11 multiple personality patients and 11 controls matched for age and sex, Putnam et al. (1982) compared the visual evoked potentials (VEPs) of alter egos, and those of simulated alternate personalities. The VEPs were to four intensities of light and were recorded from leads placed at the vertex and occiput, with the right ear as a reference. Using Fisher's (1958) method of intraclass correlation coefficients, Putnam found no significant differences between the simulated personalities of the controls. However, the alter egos of the patients had significantly lower correlations in the heights of the peaks (amplitude) and in their location (latency). Putnam cautiously concludes that although the data suggest that normals are not able to "fake" this condition, a study using professional actors might produce different results. He also raises the possibility that the differences in VEPS may not reflect underlying neurophysiological differences but simply a systematic artefact generated by some of the patients' alter egos.

In their study of Faith, Larmore, Ludwig and Cain (1977) also noted major differences in the amplitudes and latencies of VEPs across personalities. These authors concluded that the differences "were such as would be expected if four separate individuals had been tested."

Larmore et al. (1977) found no significant differences between personalities in electrocardiograms, galvanic skin response, or blood pressure. However, Bahnson and Smith (1975) noted that alternate personalities evidenced major changes in heart rate, respiratory pauses and GSR in a *single* case followed over 8 months of therapy.

The most thorough single case study is that of Jonah (Ludwig et al., 1972) whose headaches and alpha blocking have already been mentioned. Ludwig et al. report definite qualitative differences in VEPs such that those in "Sammy" and "Usoffa" were prominent and similar, none were obtained from "King Young" and only a small potential was recorded from Jonah. Also measured were the GSRs of the four personalities to emotionally laden words. Each personality provided a number of such words and two of these were selected for each personality by the investigators. These were then randomly interspersed with 12 neutral words thus providing a standard list of 20 words. It was found that all alter egos reacted to Jonah's two words, even more so than Jonah himself. Otherwise, GSR deflections tended to be specific in that each of the other three personalities reacted only to its own pair of words. It seemed as if Jonah alone shared his affects with the other personalities.

A thorough neurological examination provoked no abnormalities nor between-personality differences save for the finding that Usoffa had reduced two-point discrimination and pain sense which was consistent with clinical interview information that he was immune to pain.

To examine the extent of amnesia or learning transfer effects among personalities, three memory tasks were performed; paired words, and the paired-associate learning and logical memory subtests of the Wechsler Memory Scale (Wechsler, 1945). In the paired words task four stem-lists of ten words were paired with five easy and five difficult associates. Each personality was taught one list of associations to a criterion of three perfect trials. The other three personalities would then be tested on each list. Finally, the original personality was retested on his "own" list to check for spontaneous memory loss. Although all personalities gained almost perfect scores when retested in this way, they fared very badly when tested on the lists of other personalities which Ludwig et al. interpret as evidence that "there is virtually no transfer of memory from any other personality to the other three."

On the paired-associate learning sub-test, Jonah was first given three trials until there was complete learning. The list was then given to the other three personalities. The second form of the test was then given first to Usoffa, and then in a different order to the other personalities. The results point to a clear practice effect across personalities but, curiously, Ludwig et al. regard this as a dramatic finding, exclaiming, "in other words, material learned by one personality facilitates learning by the subsequent personalities tested!." The authors seem to have missed the point. What would be more interesting would be an absence of such practice effects given the imputed separateness of the personalities. A sceptical position predicts just such an outcome whether it be called facilitation, practice effect, generalisation or "personality leakage" (Ludwig et al.).

Even greater practice effects across personalities were noted in the logical memory task which requires cold recall of a prose passage along the lines of a news item. They noted a similar generalisation on the Kohs blocks subtest of the Wechsler Adult Intelligence Scale.

Their explanation of the discrepancy between these findings and the absence of transfer in the paired-words task runs as follows: "Unlike the [Wechsler] Associate Learning task, where corrective feedback takes place after each trial, the ten paired words are overlearned or mastered at first by one personality and then the ten stem words are presented to each subsequent personality for its associations (without corrective feedback) to them. In a real sense, this represents a word association test, which is well known to be sensitive to personality and emotional factors." They go on to argue that the personalities do not share emotional experiences with each other hence the absence of transfer.

However, this is unacceptable ad hoc theorising. The paired word task is first presented as a test of memory, and then, after producing discrepant results, gets retranslated into an affect-laden word association task. (In fact, some generalisation was evident but only from Jonah to the other personalities, as with the GSRs. This is described, rather than explained, as deriving from the other personalities' access to Jonah's psyche, but not to each other's.)

These investigators also used a classical conditioning paradigm using electric shock to the calf as the unconditioned stimulus (UCS). A different conditioned stimulus (CS) was presented to each personality comprising tones of 600 Hz and 1200 Hz, a flashing light and opening of a hand. A positive GSR was taken as the conditioned response provided it was greater than the baseline GSR to the original UCS. Each personality was then exposed to all the CS. Hypalgesic Usoffa failed to condition much at all and the remaining results are described by the authors as "inconsistent and confusing". For all that, the results do show considerable generalisation across personalities. King Young and Sammy, for example, responded to all CS and Jonah to all but that of Usoffa.

In their final comments they say they can conceive of "no way that these results, taken in total, could have been produced solely through the mechanisms of deception or intense role-playing, or both, even though these mechanisms may have been operative to some degree." It is, none the less, worth reiterating that there is more to the "problem of multiple personality" than choosing between "reality" and faking. Let the last words on their paper be the authors. "All individuals, to some extent, can be "different" people under different circumstances ... perhaps it is not too presumptuous to presume that all individuals, no matter how well adjusted, have at least a touch of multiple personality within them."

Braun (1983) has documented a number of "alternate-specific" physiological responses citing three cases where personalities exhibited allergies and a further three cases who produced dermatological reactions. He also refers to a case with an alternate-specific seizure disorder, and a patient who "passed pain" around among her personalities until the pain threshold of each personality was reached. Finally, he notes that multiple personality patients appear to heal more rapidly than non-multiples (Braun and Braun, 1979; Allison, Caul and Kluft, personal communications). Given that such phenomena are known to be susceptible to hypnosis he posits, in line with Bliss (e.g. 1986) that a form "of hypnosis/autohypnosis may be a common denominator (although) the question of the neurophysiologic effect of hypnotic suggestion has not as yet been studied with appropriate controls or safeguards."

Although the continuing research into the physiological aspects of this phenomenon may illuminate some of the underlying mechanisms and foster theory building it is unlikely to dispel the sceptic's concern. Putnam (1984) has rightly observed that the "implicit question in all of the research to date has been: 'Is it real?' Given the sensational claims often made about this disorder, this is an appropriate question. It is a question, however, that is extremely difficult to answer based on psychophysiologic data. At the present time there is not a single measure or combination of measures that can reliably establish the existence of any psychiatric diagnostic category."

The same can be said of investigations using psychological tests although they, too, may cast some indirect light on this problem. It is to these few researches that we now turn.

The first objective study of a multiple personality was that of Morton Prince (1906) who employed McDougall's categorisation of the emotions to study Miss Beauchamp.

A considerably more sophisticated study was that of Osgood and Luria (1954). At the suggestion of McV. Hunt, at that time the editor of the *Journal of Abnormal and Social Psychology*, Thigpen and Cleckley administered the semantic differential (Osgood, 1952) to their patient, Eve. Osgood and Luria (1954) then subjected the resultant protocols to a blind analysis.

The semantic differential is essentially a simple clinical tool which requires the subject to allocate a given element to a point on a continuum bounded by bipolar constructs. In this respect it resembles the Repertory Grid Test associated with Kelly's Theory of Personal Constructs (Kelly, 1955). Osgood found many of the scales were highly intercorrelated and a factor analysis revealed three general factors under which most continua could be subsumed, namely, "evaluation", "potency", and "activity." Examples would be, "kind-cruel", "strong-weak" and "active-passive." In the form administered to Eve, 15 elements were rated against 10 such bipolar constructs yielding a 1510 matrix. Osgood (1954) explains that the meaning of a particular concept to the subject ... is the profile of numbers in its column (or, more efficiently, the position in the n-dimensional space defined by the projection of these numbers onto the factors. Difference in meaning for two concepts is defined by the distance between their positions in this space, as computed by the generalized distance formula, $D = \sqrt{\Sigma d^2}$, in which d is the difference in allocation of the two concepts on a single scale. The more similar any two concepts are in connotative meaning, the smaller will be the value of D. Change in meaning (of the same concept at different times during therapy, or in different "personalities") can be defined by the same operation, except that d here refers to the differences in allocation of the same concept on the same scale at different testings. The mathematical properties of this formula also allow us to represent the semantic structure of an individual in a concise form; computation of the distance, D, of every concept from every other concept yields an N/N matrix (here15/15) of distances which have the property of plotting within a space having dimensionality equal to the number of factors. To the extent that the individual subject being studied uses the same three general factors isolated factorially, his or her data will plot accurately in three dimensions.

Eve was tested twice in each personality, with a 2-month interval between testings. Osgood and Luria then produced character sketches of the three personalities. Thus Eve White emerged as socialised, construing the world "normally", but had an unsatisfactory attitude toward herself; Eve Black had "achieved a violent kind of adjustment", saw herself as perfect and perceived the world "abnormally"; Jane emerged as having the most "healthy" perception of the world and the most satisfactory self-evaluation. They also noted that Eve Black's construct system was the least stable over time, and the least internally consistent.

The correlations of each personality with itself was regularly higher than the correlations between personalities (save for Eve White and Jane on the first testing) which the authors saw as quantitative justification for stating that the semantic differential did distinguish between the different personalities. Osgood and Luria go on to be more speculative and even "rhapsodic" (their own adjective) about the three personalities but are explicit that their hunches about possible dynamics and prognosis depart from the factual data and are distinct from the objective aspects of their study.

Although frankly acknowledging that this analysis was "merely (putting) into words what (Eve had) indicated by her check marks", Osgood was encouraged by its accuracy. However, it was more than twenty years before we learn that he was given the opportunity to conduct another blind analysis (Osgood et al., 1976). The invitation came from Jeans whose patient presented with three personalities, Gina, Mary and Evelyn. On this occasion, the semantic differential was administered only once, and 25 elements were rated using the same 10 constructs as previously. Once again, Osgood acknowledges that the emergent characterisations were "little more than verbalisations of the information provided by the patient in her scale-checking behaviour" (Osgood et al., 1976) but Jeans (1976) was none the less impressed by their accuracy as well as by the speculations by Osgood et al. about ethnic, economic and family structure and their surmise that the patient's sister had married against her mother's wishes. However, it is clear from Jeans' paper (curiously published, along with that of Osgood et al., not until 10 years after the test administration in 1967) that his predictions and interpretations were not always at one with the semantic differential data. Instead, he accommodates the objective findings into his scheme of things using ad hoc explanations and referring to his own scepticism in the clinical setting. For example he says of Gina that, "too often I thought that she did not really mean what she was saying and that she was merely using an exaggerated way of expressing herself. She wasn't. The exaggeration was Gina."

Another example of what seems a most tendentious congruence can be seen in the following quote from Jeans: "Another reason why my predictions were slightly inaccurate in regard to Evelyn is that I predicted according to what I thought her reactions would be if SEX and MY SPOUSE (two of the rated elements) became realities for her, as indeed they did shortly after the tests were completed. Her responses reflected where she was at the time of testing ... I am fairly sure that her responses ... would be different now that she is happily married." Jeans leaves one in no doubt about his willingness to compromise rather than objectively evaluate when he concludes, "As to the comparative validity of intimate clinical versus remote objective interpretation, I have learned as a result of this experience that they are complementary, and that there is nothing to lose and much to be gained by their complementarity. The pressure of practice and a certain confidence in my clinical ability had prevented me from drawing as much meaning from my data as I could when confronted with the results of the blind analysis."

Despite the attractiveness of Jeans' undogmatic eclecticism such a position hampers clear conclusions about the validity of either his clinical judgements or this particular objective assessment.

In their study of Jonah, Ludwig et al. (1972), included the Adjective Check List (ACL) of Gough and Heilbrun (1965), a Draw-Self Task, intelligence measures comprising the Kent Emergency Scale, the Shipley Institute of Living Scale and the WAIS Similarities and Block Design subtests, and the MMPI (Short Form - R). We are told that detailed analysis of the ACL results was not feasible and the summary observation was made that Usoffa was the most different, and Sammy and King Young were the most similar, whilst all four personalities evidenced little motivation for change. Of the Draw-Self Task data, the authors say that "the reader's interpretations are just as valid as our own." So far, then, one might wonder why these tasks were chosen. The former admits no analysis. The latter is open to all-comers for interpretation. The presentation of the results of the intelligence measures are similarly bland . The "raw scores ... indicate that all personalities possess a roughly similar IQ" (Ludwig et al., 1972).

On the MMPI, all personalities were similar on K (validity), Hs (Hypochondriasis), Pt (Psychasthenia), D (Depression) and Ma (Mania). This they paraphrase as "some ego-resources, no somatic symptoms or discomfort, generally pleasant and outgoing but impulsive under stress." Jonah emerged as the most willing to admit his problems (F-K index; Gough, 1950) and Sammy as the most prone to answer in the socially desirable direction (high L). Jonah's profile was described as "chronic paranoic schizophrenic." The authors go on to say that his thinking was over-inclusive tending towards a "sawtooth" profile, and exhibited High Sc, F and Pa. They note that F is sensitive to schizophrenia, is uncorrelated with the neurotic, hysteric scales, Hs and Hy (Hysteria), and "in this context is usually indicative of a borderline state used to control frank psychosis." Evidence for the latent Usoffa is seen in the peaks on Pa

(Paranoia), Sc (Schizophrenia), Pd (Psychopathic Deviation) and Ma which they interpret as pointing to the possibility of sudden aggressive behaviour.

Brandsma and Ludwig felt that the consistency of the results pointed away from the possibility of conscious faking by a "lower-class, intellectually normal patient." They conclude that multiple personalities are unique entities lying outside current, conceptual schema. "They are not clearly psychotic, neurotic, hysteric or schizophrenic (but) combine aspects of many traditional syndromes."

Bliss (1984) also has produced MMPI data on 15 female patients meeting the DSM III criteria for multiple personality and states that a relatively consistent profile emerged. However, although he found elevations on F (Validity) and Sc, similar to those of Jonah, there were also elevations on every other scale, save the two validity scales, L and K. The clinical utility of such data is questionable. It is hard to see how they might be interpreted or aid in differential diagnosis. Bliss's (1984) closing comments on these results does not conflict with this view. He writes, "there should be multiples, those with a lesser number of symptoms, who do not show this profile, and there should be others with this profile who are not multiples."

Finally, there have been studies employing the Rorschach test. Here I refer to those of Wagner and Heise (1974) and of Danesino et al. (1979) although the results of other investigations using this projective technique will be found elsewhere in this monograph in the context of particular cases. At the outset it should be noted that the Rorschach is a controversial test. Eysenck (1958) regards this test as of no demonstrable value whatsoever and Vernon (1964) believes that "projective techniques ... are one of the major issues that divide the clinically orientated from the psychometric psychologist." Lord (1950) has shown that the order of testing, wording of instructions and even the personality of the tester can significantly affect Rorschach responses. Indeed the training of the test administrator, the edition of the blots, and even the lighting have all been implicated as significant situational determinants of responses to this test.

Wagner (1971) has proposed a theory of personality called Structural Analysis (SA) which posits two complementary and reciprocal structures, the Facade Self (FS) and the Introspective Self (IS). Briefly, the FS is reality orientated and preverbal in origin whilst the IS is concerned with the establishment of a self-concept and the evolution of a fantasy life, and is dependent upon language. "The FS reacts, the IS attempts to interact. The FS is environmentally programmed while the IS is self-programmed" (Wagner, 1971). An extensively developed IS imposed on a weak FS would lead to schizoid personality formation. Conversely, a poorly developed IS together with rigid attempts at buttressing the FS is hypothesised as producing coping mechanisms such as "professionalisation" (identifying with one's work), "sexualisation" (providing proof of one's sexual identity through clothes and overtly sexual behaviour) and "socialisation" (joining clubs and societies). Dissociation and repression, in this scheme, represent less efficient attempts at coping with a weak FS.

Wagner deduces that Form (F) and Colour (C) Rorschach responses are manifestations of the FS whereas movement responses reveal IS tendencies. "Light shading (chiaroscuro) responses associated with F responses reflects difficulty in expressing FS tendencies in the face of environmental constraints: shading which appears in conjunction with movement determinants reflects concern with the discharge of IS impulses" (Wagner, 1971). For a fuller account of Wagner's thesis the reader is referred to Wagner and Heise (1974) and Wagner (1981).

In their study of the Rorschach protocols of three multiple personality cases, Wagner and Heise (1974) found a large number of movement responses both in absolute and percentage terms, together with colour responses which were inconsistent and oppositional. In a later study (Wagner, 1978) of a patient diagnosed as an hysterical fugue state, a similar pattern of responses was found. Wagner notes that the term "fugue state" was used in the classical sense to denote "the intrusion into consciousness of an alien personality capable of operating independently over time and producing a reason for flight."

Danesino et al. (1979) studied a 26-year-old female presenting with four personalities. The primary personality was called Jo-Jo and initially complained of depression, fatigue, suicidal thoughts and inability to deal with a recent childbirth. She also complained of memory lapses and reported dreams of waking to find herself with her hands around her neck. She was passive, intellectual and compulsive with sexual conflicts. A second personality, Josephine was hedonistic, loud and sexually uninhibited. The third personality, Baby Jo-Jo, behaved like a 3 year old, sucking her thumb and rolling on the floor. The fourth personality, Joanne, appeared some 5 months into therapy. She was confused, anxious and suicidal. The authors write that, "She did not know her name, where she was, or what was happening ... Dr Daniels gave her the name of Joanne and this seemed to relieve some of her anxiety." The Rorschach was given to Josephine, Jo-Jo and Joanne, in that order. It was not possible to obtain a record from Baby Jo-Jo, nor could a full record be obtained from Joanne whose anxiety led her to keep on running away from the test sessions. Danesino et al. found 5 and 9 movement responses in the protocols of Jo-Jo and Josephine respectively, constituting 31% and 57% of the total responses which they interpret as being consistent with the findings of Wagner and Heise (1974). The range of results they find compatible is clearly wide. In the case of Joanne there were only two movement responses but this inconsistency is explained as owing to her "overwhelming anxiety and deep regression." In line with Wagner and Heise they found a normal percentage of F responses in the case of Jo-Jo and Joanne but Josephine's protocol showed low F%. Once again, inconsistent results are quickly dealt with by Danesino et al. who refer to Josephine's "extended" (sic) F% score which moves from an initial 6.35% to 63%.

These authors refer to the issue of the credibility of multiple personality and report that "each psychogram portrays a unique and consistent structure which represents a distinct personality. A comparison of the three protocols by blind judges substantiated the reliability of this finding. Thus the credibility of the phenomenon is supported by the present study and the simulation hypothesis is rejected." This is scientific reporting at its blandest only to be matched by the comments of Danesino et al. on the possibility that multiple personality is iatrogenic: "even if direct or indirect suggestions had been advanced by the therapist and accepted by the patient, the suggestions could only have tapped previously existing hidden facets of her psychic organisation." Such statements are dogma rather than science.

The small number of cases, the absence of controls, the subjectivity of scoring procedures, the ad hoc rationalisation of inconsistent results, the incompleteness of some of the protocols as well as the reports of the experimental procedures suggest a degree of caution in evaluating the usefulness of Rorschach testing in this context.

I conclude this chapter on objective approaches by presenting the theoretical position of Oakley and Eames, from University College, London, and of Braun. The phenomenon of multiple personality has received scant attention from British researchers and clinicians but a noteworthy exception is a paper by Oakley and Eames (in Oakley ed., 1985) entitled "The Plurality of Consciousness". They begin by suggesting that we may be mistaken in our everyday impression of the unified nature of consciousness. A model of human awareness is proposed where the subcortex (dealing with simple reflexes, homeostasis and association learning) is surrounded by cortical systems "devoted to forming inner representations of the real world." These systems are the dynamic basis for "internal experimentation ... reasoning and insight ... for storing information from experience as a biographical record. This personal history, or episodic memory, retains events in spatially and temporally coded form." Informational stores are abstracted from the ongoing stream of consciousness and, freed from spatial and temporal context, constitute semantic memory. We are, however, also aware of ourselves as actors in the world and can reflect on the contents of consciousness so that we are aware both of our perceptions of the external environment as well as our own inner feelings and evaluations. Thus it is posited that there exists "a separate cortical system superimposed on the cortical representational systems of each hemisphere" and this is responsible for selecting samples of representations from consciousness for "rerepresentation within a system of priority processing." Nothing, therefore, can enter self-awareness if it has not first entered consciousness. It is well established, for example, that Pavlovian conditioning is mediated by non-conscious association processes.

This does not imply, however, that all that enters consciousness necessarily enters self-awareness. A common example is the phenomenon of subliminal perception where it has been demonstrated that the meaning of stimuli, presented at sub-threshold levels and unavailable to introspection, can affect percepts, verbal report and emotional responses (e.g. Dixon, 1981; Dixon and Henley, 1980). Oakley also cites the putative influence of pheromones on behaviour (Keverne, 1983) and the Poetzl effect where aspects of a stimulus configuration which are not consciously perceived have demonstrable influence on descriptions of later dream content. Relatedly, anaesthetised patients have shown an ability to recall, under hypnosis, dialogues between their surgeon and the aneasthetist (Levinson, 1965, cited in Cheek and LeCron, 1968). A mundane example of that which enters consciousness but not self-awareness are the many routine behaviours which underlie everyday life such as switching off lights when leaving a room or changing gear whilst driving.

The human brain, of course, comprises two hemispheres and although there is some truth in the maxim that "two heads are better than one" there can also be disadvantages. Which (or who) is to be the originator of any particular required action? Two can be a crowd since there is room for competition as well as cooperation.

Split-brain patients can discover that the right hand literally does not know what the left hand is doing, and Oakley and Eames cite Dimond's (1979) account of such a patient who found their left hand, "as if with a mind of its own", reaching out to prevent their right hand picking something up. Interestingly, it is observed that (in right-handed patients) the right hand (under left hemisphere control) is typically regarded as being "me" whilst the left hand is seen as the obstructing alien. Nor do patients report any change in the subjectively experienced self following commisurectomy or even entire removal of the right hemisphere. However, Oakley and Eames note that "what is missing after such surgical interventions is the ability of the left, speaking hemisphere to directly access representations within consciousness systems in the right hemisphere." This, in turn, leads to affectively blunted speech, impoverishment of emotional experience and fewer reported dreams.

There is also evidence that the right hemisphere can not only represent itself within consciousness but also has an established biographical and general information store (e.g. LeDoux et al., 1979; Sperry et al., 1979). Oakley and Eames express the cerebral relationship nicely when they write:

> The left hemisphere acts as "spokesman" for the split-brain individual, and provides as plausible an account as possible for the individual's behaviour. There seems to us no reason to suppose that the same should not be true of intact brains, and that many of the indecisions, inspirations and "unaccountable" mood changes about which our left hemispheres rationalise are consequences of conscious processes within our right hemispheres. Clearly, if the reactions of two connected hemispheres to similar situations are too divergent, mental pathology may result. It is perhaps no coincidence that the majority of psychosomatic symptoms appear on the left side of the body, possibly as the right hemisphere, denied a verbal outlet, finds its own means of communicating its distress.

These authors point out the inadequacy of explaining multiple personality merely as the alternation between hemispheres of executive control of two self-awareness systems. Apart from reports of a multiplicity of alter-egos "the personal history and self-representation in the hemisphere with a suppressed self-awareness system are very similar to those of the dominant hemisphere. An alternation between these two systems would result in two rather similar personalities with a common life history." Instead they suggest that the normal individual adopts a diversity of roles during development. As a rule these roles are seen as integrated aspects of the same self-representation. However, in the case of multiple personality a childhood trauma causes a sudden role shift of such proportions that a the new self-representation is now read as a discrete entity. Henceforth, a new set of episodic memories is generated which are inaccessible to the primary personality, although limited information transfer is possible between susbsystems. For Oakley and Eames, multiple personality is not a case of different selves being continually recreated (by, for example, situational demands or radical mood changes). Rather, they conceive of all subsystems as concurrently active and any given set of behaviours and subjective experience are dependent upon which particular self-representation is being read into the self-awareness system at any given time; in other words, "'We' experience what our consciousness systems decide to re-represent in self-awareness."

In sum, their model posits that "multiple parallel streams of conscious activity ... present in normal individuals ... can be attached to different self-representations, and so when re-presented are revealed as the thoughts of different individuals ... our unitary perspective of our own conscious processes is a consequence of the constraints imposed by our viewing them through the limited window of self awareness." They also subscribe to an anatomical rather than functional distinctiveness between the separate subsystems despite acknowledging that neurological studies have so far failed to support such a thesis.

The model of Oakley and Eames is at a conspicuously early stage of development and despite the grounding of their constructs in the language of neurophysiology and information technology one wonders whether they are really providing fresh insights. Is there a radical difference between the, previously encountered, notion of "ego-states" with more-or-less permeable boundaries and Oakley and Eames' subsystems of self-representation with varying degrees of "memory blockade" between them? Perhaps Oakley's most helpful contribution in this context is the distinction he draws between "consciousness" and "self-awareness" and, as he rightly says, a split-brain operation on a multiple personality patient would be most illuminating.

Braun (1984) has proposed a complex and eclectic theory which attempts to subsume the phenomena of multiple personality under the rubric of state-dependent learning (SDL). SDL refers to the fact that things learned in a particular environment, or in a particular physiological state are frequently best recalled when that state is recreated. In other words, the original learning environment serves as a recall cue, something which Tulving (1978) has termed "encoding specificity". Police investigations make use of this notion when they arrange the re-enactment of a crime at the original scene using look-alike actors. This procedure frequently triggers off memories from witnesses who previously failed to recall any of the details of the crime. Similarly, things learned in a mildly intoxicated state may sometimes only be recalled when the individual is again intoxicated.

Learning theories of SDL argue that learning leads to changes in the perception of internal and external contemporaneous cues. Research from animal discriminatory drug learning suggests that memories are only available for retrieval when the drug is reintroduced into the nervous system of the animal to recreate or associate to the original encoding cues.

Neuroanatomic theories posit the creation of new cell assemblies during learning and drugs cause their reactivation. Drugs may also induce an alteration in neuronal excitability, sensitivity, or output that must be recreated by the drug for the memory to be recalled (Braun, 1984).

Task complexity, sleep, circadian rhythm and mood states have all been implicated in SDL. For example, Braun cites one of Weingartner's (1976) experiments where his subjects were hypnotically induced to be either "happy" or "sad" and then instructed to engage in free recall. He found that happy subjects recalled more happy memories (92%) and sad subjects, more sad memories (55%), pointing to mood-dependent recall. Further clinical support for this thesis is the frequent natural occurrence of SDL in manic-depressive patients.

Braun observes that dissociation can occur under extreme stress and suggests that a possible mechanism, secondary to ACTH-endorphin release, is excess from arcuate nucleus cells which change the noradrenalin/serotonin balance from the locus ceruleus and raphe. The subsequent disconnection of the cortex would lead to the limbic system, and more primitive emotional responses being given priority. Repeated dissociations under stress (e.g. child abuse) could facilitate the formation of discrete personalities via SDL. The reinforcement for such SDL could be the drop in ACTH level when the stress is reduced. In this way, alternate personalities might be conceptualised as dissociated "software programs". Braun speculates that the switching between personalities is dependent on a classically conditioned (probably limbic, ACTH-facilitated) process. Operant conditioning and reinforcement would then maintain these alternate modes of self-expression. There is more to Braun's model, drawing on what he terms "cellular learning"; peptide research; the creation of holograms via slow-wave fields, optics and Bentov's (1977) esoteric theory that human beings (and, indeed all matter) are "standing waves of 'sound' vibratory energy." All but the kitchen sink appears in Braun's paper, including Miller, Galanter and Pribram's (1960) Test-Operate-Test-Exit (TOTE) model which proposed a feedback information-processing loop whereby stimulus inputs are matched against internal tenplates to ensure "goodness of fit". Braun suggests that the multiple personality patient has several "monitor images" (personalities) against which to match inputsand this leads to the longevityof the personalities. Normal individuals have only one "monitor image" (personality) and, therefore, behave more or less consistently because their TOTE system will modify behaviour and experience (via anxiety) which threatens disequilibrium. Braun's approach is frankly speculative and the sweep of its eclecticism is as clever as it is daunting. So far, however, no one has taken up the gauntlet to develop his synthesis further.

CHAPTER 6

Multiple Personality, Hypnosis and Dissociation

Comparisons between hypnosis and multiple personality have a long history, dating back to the work of Janet (1889, 1907) and Prince (1906).

Perhaps the most obvious common denominator is that both seem to include what Ludwig (1966) has termed "altered states of consciousness" (ASCs). During ASCs there is a significant deviation from normal alertness so that individuals become more than usually preoccupied with internal processes, both physiological and mental, and there is a suspension in reality testing in favour of more "autistic" modes of thinking. The former is frequently characterised as a more active, and explicitly goal-directed or problem-solving activity. Autistic thinking, on the other hand, is characterised by a passive, receptive mental state, allowing more scope to fantasy and creative thinking. Doubtless, creative activities use both thinking modes sequentially, an initial period where imagination is given free rein followed by an explicitly critical, "editing" operation.

Current attitudes to this, doubtless oversimplified, dichotomy locate reality orientated thinking in the left hemisphere, with the right hemisphere being primarily concerned with more autistic processes (e.g. Hilgard, 1977).

Ludwig (1966) suggests five sets of circumstances that can produce ASCs.

Firstly, there are situations where sensory input is drastically reduced as occurs, for example, in solitary confinement, during prolonged periods at sea or in the desert, following bilateral cataract operations, or in experimental sensory deprivation states.

Secondly, ASCs can be a consequence of sensory bombardment or "overload", such as might be experienced during "brainwashing" or "third degree" interrogation techniques, mob violence, or religious rites of the kind described by Sargant in his book, *Battle For The Mind* (1957). Sargant imputed the ecstatic trance states sometimes seen during religious conversion ceremonies to acute overarousal leading to what he termed "transmarginal inhibition". Ludwig argues that ASCs can also be produced by excessive "inner emotional turbulence or conflict secondary to external conditions conducive to heightened emotional arousal."

Third, are those conditions of increased alertness or mental involvement as when individuals are required to be especially vigilant for long periods, for example, scanning radar screens. Similarly, ASCs may result from the prolonged focusing of attention on a particular stimulus configuration such as the sound of a metronome, a charismatic speaker or a book in which one is mentally absorbed.

At the other end of the spectrum are the fourth set of conditions when individuals suspend focused, active thinking, as in meditation, reverie, deep relaxation or "free associative states during psychoanalytic therapy."

Finally, Ludwig refers to somatopsychological factors which may be physiological disturbances such as changes in blood sugar level, hyperventilation or temporal lobe seizures. There are also ASCs which are the direct consequence of pharmacological agents, notably the hallucinogens.

Ludwig summarises the general characteristics of the resultant ASCs as follows. Individuals experience alterations in thinking, especially logical reasoning, and have a disturbed sense of time. They experience a sense of loss of control and demonstrate changes in the expression of emotion, often experiencing extreme mood swings and/or affective blunting. Changes in body image and depersonalisation, as well as perceptual distortions, may occur. Individuals may suddenly attach special significance or meaning to experiences and events so that they are deluded into believing they have achieved some special insight or achieved an earth-shattering solution to a profound philosophical problem. Such states are common in manic episodes. Typically, individuals will claim an inability to communicate the essence of their experience to those who have not had similar experiences. Ludwig calls this their "sense of the ineffable". Occasionally, ASCs will also include feelings of rejuvenation. Perhaps as a cumulative result of these features of ASCs, the suspension of critical thinking, the changes in emotional and perceptual experience, and the sense of profound insight, individuals also tend to be hypersuggestible.

As Ludwig puts it, "Contradictions, doubts, inconsistencies and inhibitions tend to diminish ... and the suggestions of the person endowed with authority tend to be accepted as concrete reality. These suggestions become imbued with even more importance and urgency owing to the increased significance and meaning attributed both to internal and external stimuli during alterations in consciousness."

Although Ludwig makes no allusion to multiple personality, choosing to make frequent reference to hypnotic states, it is clear that the reported subjective experiences of multiples also have much in common with ASCs.

A more explicit comparison between multiple personality and hypnosis can be found in a thoughtful paper by Gruenewald (1984). She begins by positing dissociation as a feature common to both and credits Hilgard (1977) with its contemporary revival as a useful explanatory concept. Whatever refinements may be introduced into a "theory" of dissociation the phenomenon itself is beguilingly easy to describe. This is largely because all of us experience, to a greater or lesser degree, frequent dissociative experiences throughout our lives. Apart from the, presumably rare, occasions when we are hypnotised or amnesic, we have all become "lost" in a play at the theatre or found ourselves embarrassed by an interlocutor who exposes the fact that our "minds have wandered" when they ask, "so what do you think about all I've been saying?" A serious problem for Road Research Scientists is the problem of "highway hypnosis" (Moseley, 1953) when the tedium of driving allows intrusive hypnagogic imagery to distract our attention from the task in hand. There can be few drivers who have not found themselves at a point on their journey with no recollection of the previous couple of miles. It is hardly necessary to rehearse much further everyday examples of this human propensity. In some mysterious fashion, part of us sometimes "splits off" from the rest, occasionally indulging in the most vivid fantasies, whilst "the rest" gets on quite impressively with the focus of conscious awareness. I am reminded of a tutorial with an undergraduate who began by announcing that he had recently given up smoking. He went on to elaborate with an account of his previous heavy consumption and boasted that he still carried a pack of twenty cigarettes in his pocket to prove to himself his strength of resolve. To my unkind amusement, my student's proud account was accompanied by his oblivious removal of a cigarette from his pocket, his lighting of it, and several deep inhalations before he too saw the humour of the situation. However, so fleeting may be these cognitions, and so impressive is the management of our behaviour during such everyday dissociations that the onlooker is typically unaware of such autistic "lapses."

A central problem for the theorist trying to understand the phenomenon of multiple personality is that none has yet come up with a satisfactory explanation of what "personality" means. An apocryphal tale tells of a graduate student who took over a seminar series on "Theories of Personality" when the normal lecturer, his supervisor, fell ill. On his return, a term later, the lecturer asked the student how far through the course his student had progressed. How many theories had been articulated? The student–lecturer confided that they had not yet actually got to grips with any particular theory. He and his students were still grappling with the problem of what was meant by "Personality"! One can only respect the student's good intent and one can readily understand the reaction of his supervisor who confided that he never indulged in such "semantic niceties." "Leave all that to the philosophers," he advised, "I always start straight in with Freud, Jung and Adler, and move on through Allport, Cattell and Eysenck." Such pragmatism at least has the merit that such courses get finished. However, the more inquisitive students might be forgiven for feeling somewhat bewildered by the disparity of the approaches they had encountered.

From the Radical Behaviourist position, of course, the concept of "Personality" is quite unnecessary. From this viewpoint Behaviour is a rather accidental affair and if one must use the term "Personality" it can refer to no more than one's current response repertoire deriving from a precarious history of differential reinforcement. (Some theorists admit also the role of certain, proscribed physiological factors.)

What strikes the more "dynamic" theorist is the seeming consistency of Personality.

Adults do not appear to change radically from day to day either to themselves or to the onlooker. On those few occasions when this rule of "self-consistency" seems to be broken we are most adept at explaining away our dissonant cognitions. The most cursory inspection of our manner of coping with such unpredictability reveals how tightly we hold on to an implicit faith in the unity of personality. "She's not herself today," we argue; "He's acting out of character,"; "I probably misunderstood what she meant,"; "He's only pretending"; "It's just a role that she's adopting." Or we may impute the apparent change to illness, as when we say, "He'll be back to his old self when he's well again." Professionals, too, are accustomed to suspect that radical personality changes indicate underlying pathology of an organic nature (e.g. a dementing process).

Gordon Allport's (1961) solution to this problem is to propose a hierarchical organisation of personality. In his scheme, some traits ("cardinal" traits) are much more central than others. These represent enduring dispositions and are in stark contrast to lower order traits, or habits, where flux and change are frequently evident. The recognition of these, "higher order", cardinal traits helps us to "make sense" of apparent inconsistencies in ourselves as well as in others. If someone's cardinal trait is to please others (perhaps through fear of rejection) we are likely to see them forming alliances with radically different people, to be expressing agreement with radically contrasting viewpoints.

Use of the term "dissociation", however, takes as axiomatic a model of personality where the impression of unity can be illusory. "Personality" is seen as multifaceted even to the point of comprising many different "selves", let alone different habits, values, attitudes and interests. *Inter alia*, theorists have proposed Id, Ego, and Superego; Child, Parent, and Adult; Systems of Personal Constructs; Hierarchies of Needs; and Constellations of Traits, but all are finally confronted with the problem of the overall executor, the supreme "knower" (to borrow the term used by Gordon Allport in his book, *Becoming* 1955).

However, who (or what) is it that is responsible for the coordination of all these aspects of what we call "personality"? What is the source of decision making, of behavioural selection, of that part of us that is so readily able to detach itself from all else and look on, like a spectator at a play? How can we account for that distinctively human capacity for self-reflection, self-awareness, self-consciousness?

One must beware of making "category mistakes" when tackling such essentially psychological questions. Bannister (1968) has astutely pointed out that, all too frequently, psychological questions are given physiological answers. Using the framework of Kelly's Personal Construct Theory, he observes that physiological explanations lie outside the "range of convenience" of psychological elements in the same way that the construct, say, "tough minded-tender minded" lies outside the range of convenience of the element, "carbon paper" (but comfortably within the range of convenience of the element "political attitude"). Thus if one asks a patient, "How do you feel?", one is asking a psychological question which requires a psychological answer. A response at the appropriate level would, therefore, be something like, "I feel anxious (or "embarrassed", or "guilty" ...)." An inappropriate response would be, "My blood cholesterol level is elevated (or "my SNS is activated", "there is a deflection in my GSR" ...). Therefore, in the quest for the physiological identity of the "executor" or "supreme knower", its location in the cortex or the pineal gland is of questionable value to the psychological investigator.

The central concern of the psychologist is software rather than hardware. Neisser (1966) has expressed this view with admirable clarity:

> I do not doubt that human behaviour and consciousness depend entirely on the activity of the brain, in interaction with other physical systems ... some experimental findings have hinted that the complex molecules of RNA and DNA ... may be the substrate of memory ... but Psychology is not just something 'to do until the biochemist comes' (as I have recently heard psychiatry described) .... The task of a psychologist trying to understand human cognition is analogous to that of a man trying to understand how a computer has been programmed ... he will not care much whether his particular computer stores information in magnetic cores or in thin films; he wants to understand the program, not the 'hardware'. By the same token, it would not help the psychologist to know that memory is carried by RNA as opposed to some other medium. He wants to understand its utilisation, not its incarnation. (pp. 5-6).

Thus, however intangible and elusive concepts such as Allport's "Knower" might be, they are the necessary stock in trade of the psychologist. It is, accordingly, more useful to rephrase our earlier question about "who" or "what" is the "Knower" into, "What does the 'knower' do? What is its role? What are the distinctive characteristics of its operation?

Dissociation includes a "splitting" of the personality, varies in degree, can be more or less conscious and can operate at different levels and in different guises. Dissociation is an aspect of normal mental life but it can also be manifestly pathological. Is it possible to throw some light on that form of dissociation which characterises multiple personality?

One form that dissociation takes comprises a splitting between the affective and cognitive components of experience. In these instances, the "Knower" would seem to distance itself from the emotional contents of experience. It is precisely this form of affective–cognitive splitting that characterises the defensive mechanism of "intellectualisation".

It is a common clinical experience to hear one's patient giving a most articulate, even lofty, account of the aetiology and dynamics of their current anxieties. Highly intelligent and psychologically sophisticated patients are especially prone to serving their therapists with such "insights". Indeed, trainee therapists can be quite daunted by the apparent perspicacity of their patients to the extent of wondering what is left for them to do! Here is a patient who "knows" that his difficulty with authority figures is rooted in his own poor relationship with his father. He "recognises" that his difficulty in relating to women derives from his ambivalent sexual feelings towards his mother. He "understands" his fears about cuddling his children are nourished by infant memories of an incestuous assault by his uncle. He may even describe his "insights" in the language of formal psychoanalysis, talking about "castration anxiety", "unresolved oedipal conflicts" and "projection".

However, what will ultimately dawn on both therapist and patient (hopefully, the therapist gets there first) is that access to this knowledge has nonetheless failed to alleviate the patient's anxieties. The problems remain.

It is this "stalemate" that permits the therapist to dub such accounts as "pseudo-insights", as "intellectualisations". It may be very clever but its very cleverness is its downfall. The patient's preoccupation with prosaic, even jargonesque, description serves to divert them from coming to terms with the feeling component which is necessarily involved. "Lofty" the theorising may be, both metaphorically and literally. What the patient needs in order to change, however, is rather less involvement in the role of intellectual spectator, and considerably more in the role of active experiencer.

That great director, Alfred Hitchcock, was saying as much when he was asked for guidance about playing a scene by a famous film star. "Tell me, Hitch," pleaded the anguished star, "how should I go about performing this role? What's my motivation? What dynamics am I exploring here? What's my frame of mind?" Hitchcock's reply was succinct; "Try acting", he said.

In both hypnosis and multiple personality, the "Knower" seems, at various times, to exert and relinquish control over the rest of the personality. In hypnosis, it has been suggested (e.g. Gill and Brenman, 1959) that this core component must remain unhypnotised in order to allow it to remain in contact with objective reality. In this way, it can control the degree of trance "state" or compliance with the hypnotist's suggestions. It is the "Knower" which can decide to call a halt to proceedings when, for example, continued enactment of the hypnotised role poses serious threat. It seems highly unlikely that a hypnotised subject would remain in their "trance" if shouts of "Fire!" were to be heard through the door.

I witnessed a stage hypnotist whose subject had complied with all manner of suggestions to the point of displaying what has been called "trance logic". In this condition she had been told by the hypnotist that she would not see him sitting in the chair opposite her but, instead, would hallucinate that he was sitting in a chair placed on the far side of the stage. Following this suggestion she reported with equanimity that she could now see him in both places at once. At this point, a member of the audience suddenly shouted out that the performance was fraudulent and the subject was a confederate of the hypnotist. At this, the subject came immediately out of her reverie and announced she was no such thing and had never met the hypnotist before in her life!

Gruenewald (1984) writes:

When the central control system retreats to a more passive position and merely exercises the observing function, it resembles the phenomenon of the 'hidden observer' (Hilgard, 1977). A metaphor for covert (dissociated) self-observation which some but not all highly hypnotizable subjects can verbalise by way of 'automatic talking' (akin to automatic writing and not in conscious awareness), the hidden observer denotes the persistence at some level of knowledge about ordinary reality, in contrast to the subjectively experienced 'reality' of hypnotic consciousness.

What, however, is the equivalent of the hidden observer in multiple personality? One is tempted to suggest that it is the primary personality, which has been compared to a host who has invited guests (secondary personalities) to come to its aid. However, the analogy falls down when the primary personality is described as losing all contact with, and control over, these secondary personalities. Once invited in, these guests are not simply permitted to remain, at the host's whim, and under his constant surveillance. They take over control, come and go autonomously, and are "out of sight."

However, Gruenewald goes on to note four features which reveal that these subsystems are not absolutely independent. Whatever degree of dissociation may be present in multiple personality it is far from complete:

> First, the secondary personality subsystem sinks back into the unconscious realm with the 'return' of the primary personality. Second, if hypnosis was used to call it forth, the subsystem places itself under the hypnotist's control by allowing him/her to regulate the time of its dominance. Third, a subsystem akin to the hidden observer is found in some though not all multiple personality patients. This subsystem tends to be realistically aware of the needs and interests of the primary person or of another subsystem and can instruct the therapist what action to take – for instance, to prevent a suicide. But it has to use the therapist as the acting agent and thus lacks the executive component of the central regulatory mechanism. Furthermore, despite an apparently complete dissociation, certain aspects of the temporarily non-sentient primary personality remain functional, in that the basic 'apparatuses of primary autonomy,' the 'constitutional givens,' (Hartmann, 1939/1958, p. 104), remain available to all subsystems. Although available as basic functions, however, motility, perception, memory, the capacity for intelligent thought, etc. are drawn into and selectively utilised by anyone currently dominant subsystem.

Memory functions have a central role in both hypnosis and multiple personality but, once again, there are significant differences in the kind of forgetting and retrieval that takes place. The reported amnesia of the multiple personality patient seems to be universal, involuntary and is extremely resistant to therapeutic intervention. In hypnosis, amnesia is not an invariable consequence but depends on whether the hypnotist has issued instructions to the subject that some part, or all, of the hypnotic experience should be forgotten. Even then, subjects may fail to forget despite strong motivation to comply with such suggestions for post-hypnotic amnesia. Additionally, in contrast to the resistance of the multiple personality patient, the hypnotic subject responds readily to instructions to retrieve the hitherto forgotten material. This reversibility points to an artificiality in the dissociative processes involved in hypnosis.

Gruenewald suggests that the separate "life histories" apparent in multiple personalities actually represent secondary elaborations of the nuclear fantasies and ideas that created the original dissociation: fantasy has become reality by virtue of being externalised over time in overt behaviour, and the person then is in an altered relation to external reality.

Eventually a set of state-dependent memories is accumulated which then lend continuity to memory and experience in each altered state. Whether or not memory of historical events is veridical, the events themselves are interpreted in the light of the "other self's" needs and motives and on the basis of repeated enactment of the fantasy that there is another self. In this way, the dissociative barriers between subsystems receive continual secondary reinforcement.

Once again then, Gruenewald makes the point that the differences between hypnosis and multiple personality are as striking and important as the similarities.

She distinguishes the structure of the ego, or self, in hypnosis and multiple personality in terms of the developmental stage which has been reached. In hypnosis,it is assumed that the ego is well-formed and cohesive, with a "hypnotic part executing the hypnotist's suggestions and a non-hypnotised part ... observing the hypnotic subsystem ... (or which can) restore its usual boundaries and active control when necessary." In multiple personality, however, the splitting is conceived as being rooted in an earlier, narcissistic phase of development. "The ego in multiple personality seems to suffer from a 'basic fault' (Balint, 1968) that prevents the normal development of the central regulatory function and the coalescing of opposing psychic contents."

So, Gruenewald wants to distinguish "splitting", which she regards as an aspect of primary narcissism, from the mechanism of "dissociation" which is predicated on the existence of a cohesively integrated ego; "for nothing can be 'diss-associated' before it has been 'associated'." Using the framework of ego-psychology, she argues that the precondition for a fully integrated ego is an earlier structural stage when the organism is unable not only to differentiate "self" from "other" but also cannot distinguish between object-cathexis and identification. External objects are introjected in an "undigested" fashion and form the totality of the ego rather than being ranged alongside some superordinate self-concept which is bent on attempts to assimilate such experiences to its own essential form and structure. Rather than being an ego-defensive mechanism (since there is not yet an "ego"), splitting is regarded as the organism's primitive attempts to categorise sensory, affective and cognitive experience.

Multiple personality is seen as a fixation at this stage of development whereby the ego, instead of splitting itself from "bad" objects, splits within itself. Overwhelmed by "too numerous object identifications" (Freud, 1923), the ego finds itself incapable of their assimilation and ends up by creating a series of relatively discrete subsystems.

Gruenewald posits that, "Repression and dissociation play a complementary role in the multiple personality syndrome. Splitting inthe sense of separation of one or more sets of mental content from the mainstream of ideation and in the sense of contradictory behaviour in different states (Freud, 1938/1964) represents vertical splitting and is akin to dissociation, whereas horizontal splitting implies a separation of the reality ego from archaic levels and represents repression (Kohut, 1971)." Vertical splitting, then, refers to the compartmentalisation of current ideations and experience and bears comparison with parallel information processing. Horizontal splitting has an historical connotation and arises from the failure thus far to integrate "bad" objects because of their observed threat to the integrity of the personality.

Gruenewald notes that another distinction between these two forms of splitting, the dissociative and the repressive, is that vertical, dissociative splitting is not confined to "bad" objects. "An introject can also represent a wished-for identity, or ... potentialities which the conscious person dare not acknowledge or express, e.g. the "Victoria" personality of Sybil."

In sum then, a further distinction between hypnosis and multiple personality is that the former includes vertical, and the latter, both vertical and horizontal modes of splitting.

Finally, Gruenewald makes a brief incursion into social psychological speculation, comparing hypnosis and multiple personality in terms of role theory. Both, for example, may be seen as rule following behaviour where the rules assume compelling strength and lead to greatly restricted focusing of attention. Both may be seen as predicated on shared understandings and expectations about role performance between actor and audience (and, one might add, about just who it is who is going to be "actor" or "audience" at any given time. Both logically require that the role behaviours already exist in the repertoire of the player. However, Gruenewald sees as distinctive that, "the reality of the roles adopted by the subentities of multiple personality rests ultimately on role models encountered in the real world and in their intrapsychic representations."

This is a modest enough deduction and there seems no reason why it should not also apply to the behaviour of the hypnotic subject. The other distinction she makes is to assert that hypnotic role enactment is voluntary, despite a subjective sense of compulsion, whereas multiple personalities have relatively less control over their performances. Such an assertion counts more as an act of faith than a theoretical speculation, however.

To conclude, Gruenewald sees hypnosis and multiple personality as "sharing certain pathways but not as representing similar conditions" and with this I concur.

What then of the possibility already mooted that hypnotic procedures "cause" multiple personality? Gruenewald dismisses this likelihood, preferring to see the hypnotic situation merely as providing permission for the covert personalities to parade themselves. In her formulation, hypnosis serves to dissociate the central control system and responsibility for the emergence of alter egos is assumed by the hypnotist.

Allison (1978), in similar vein, has written, "I consider hypnosis the method by which one can open Pandora's box in which the personalities already reside. I do not believe that such hypnotic procedures create the personalities any more than the radiologist creates lung cancer when he takes the first X-rays of the chest."

Braun (1981) is also of the opinion that hypnosis cannot create multiple personality although it may be useful in its elucidation and treatment. He supports this assertion by noting Allison's (1978) report that 45% of the 30 cases he cited at that time had their first "split" before age 5, and 85% before age 10. Braun confirms that his experience was similar, stating that, "Of the 28 cases for which I have sufficient information, all had their first split before age 5, and for the vast majority, the first split occurred during the first four years of life."

Need one say that, some form of splitting (be it "horizontal," "vertical," "repressive," "dissociative," or merely gross behavioural inconsistency) surely characterises the mental lives of us all, from infancy to old age. Braun is treading a slippery conceptual slope when he implies that such "first splits" alone can be taken as evidence of the existence of multiple personality in childhood, before these individuals had been hypnotised.

Braun cites an early study by Harriman (1943), some of whose hypnotised subjects produced automatic writing and fantastic histories which Harriman took as tentative evidence that they had created another personality under hypnosis. However, despite Harriman's own caution about confusing hypnotic-role enactment with multiple personality, Braun is unreservedly dismissive: "The results of these studies ... would not surprise anyone familiar with hypnosis: to suggest that they shed light on the mechanisms of multiple personality is fanciful."

A study by Leavitt (1947) receives similar peremptory treatment from Braun although Leavitt's subject created a "bad" alter ego under hypnosis which was given a name. This study is dismissed because the personality was not sufficiently "full blown with a life history of its own." Nor, one might add, are a great many of the putative alter egos in the multiple personality literature. We have already quoted Coons (1980, 1984) who is quite frank about including under the head of "multiple personality", "states," "short-lived personalities," and "incompletely formed personality fragments."

The next study to be given short shrift by Braun is that of Kampman (1976). 41% of Kampman's highly hypnotisable subjects responded positively to a suggestion to create a secondary personality which existed before their birth. Unfortunately, Kampman does not report fully her subject's creations and Braun rightly points to the difficulty in evaluating the results of her study. Nonetheless, he cautiously concludes, "it seems wildly unlikely that her procedures produced multiple personalities by any reasonable criteria."

Thus, Gruenewald, Allison and Braun all agree that multiple personality and hypnosis are both "states", but not the same states and the latter does not cause the former. Kluft (1982) is equally sceptical that personalities can be hypnotically created.

Bliss (e.g. 1984, 1986), however, adopts a confusing position in that he unequivocally believes multiple personality is not merely the iatrogenic product of hypnotherapy yet he believes the primary underlying mechanism is self-hypnosis. Presumably, part of the ego splits off and adopts the role of external hypnotist. Further, Bliss is more than willing to acknowledge that personalities can be experimentally induced and has deliberately employed such a strategy in therapy. He tells us (Bliss, 1984) how on one occasion he "intentionally induced a new personality via hypnosis with the hope that he might be able to assist me in therapy. This was accomplished rapidly, and henceforth he could be called at will." Support for Bliss's notion comes indirectly from his observation that multiple personality patients are normally excellent hypnotic subjects, as indicated by high scores on tests of hypnotic susceptibility. More direct evidence is provided not only by their ready hypnotizability in therapy but by their proneness to "drop into trances when painful events are approached ... not only do they repeatedly and rapidly transform into these dissociated states, but some in the process of therapy have for short periods become aphonic, blind, paralysed, depersonalised, anaesthetic, and amnesic." They will also report that the experience of deep hypnosis is strikingly similar to the emergence of an alter ego. One patient explained, "In deep hypnosis you give up, are calm, totally numb, your body is relaxed, and you can't move. The next and final step is you are gone – everything is black. When Lisa (a personality) takes over, it is the same feeling."

Bliss reports that his patients date such hypnotic experiences from childhood when they fantasised about imaginary companions. He posits a continuum whereby such fantasy figures begin by being recognised as the products of their imagination and their entrances and exits are under voluntary control. With the advent of trauma, self-hypnosis is employed to create further fantasy figures to cope with the varying demands of different stressful situations. Bliss acknowledges that it is arbitrary where one draws the line between imaginary playmates and multiple personalities but says he is inclined to separate the two "at the point of partial or complete amnesia when the individual's autonomy is being compromised."

Frankel (1976) has also remarked upon the similarity between certain clinical syndromes and hypnotic states, of which multiple personality is only one. He writes:

> Occasional symptoms or clinical pictures have qualities that resemble characteristics of the trance experience. Feelings such as depersonalisation or dissociation; involuntary behaviour that is recognised as exaggerated, irrational but unavoidable such as a phobic attack; or disabling physical complaints such as pain or paresis in response to unconscious forces – all have similarities to the distorted perceptions, compelling ideas, and somatic experiences that can be introduced into hypnosis. Further clinical observation reveals that the clinical symptoms enumerated above occur in patients who are hypnotisable or highly hypnotisable.

He suggests that this hypnotisability is a relatively stable, and factorially complex attribute which is normally distributed and shows no sex differences, or trait relationships in normal populations but children are reliably more hypnotisable than adults. He also believes that there is no correlation with everyday dissociation.

He refers to a patient, Martha/Harriet, whose multiple personality he felt sure was not created by hypnotherapy because she complained of a "voice" in her head prior to consultation and hypnosis. He also says, somewhat cryptically, that the diagnostic milieu did not "favour creation" of multiple personality. Simulation is similarly ruled out when Frankel states, "there seemed little doubt ... she was caught up in a false perception rather than a game of pretence." Frankel posits that trance is a "coping mechanism" and can be deliberately employed by the therapist to break down the lines of demarcation in multiple personality patients, as well as to deal with other clinical problems. Trance, he suggests, can be used therapeutically "to create the symptoms or a facsimile of them, thereby increasing the patient's familiarity with the trance experience, on the assumption that the clinical picture was initiated by the occurrence of a spontaneous trance. In this way, a coping mechanism (can be) added to the patient's repertoire." It is possible that Frankel is describing the more familiar technique of covert, or imaginal, desensitisation although he would presumably claim that trance is a qualitatively different experience on the part of the patient. It must also be said that demonstrating the usefulness of trance in alleviating a patient's symptoms is insufficient grounds for arguing that it was trance that generated them originally.

Given that multiple personality patients seem especially hypnotisable, the question still remains as to how we account for this correlation. Such an observed consistency is an inspiration for a theory but, surely not, as Bliss seems to suggest, a theory per se. Although it is argued that early positive reinforcement, and even genetic endowment (Bliss, 1984), create a susceptibility to hypnosis which in turn can produce the syndrome of multiple personality, it might equally be argued that multiple personality is a precursor of hypnotic susceptibility. Let us imagine a child who found his/herself confronted with a body of evidence that they frequently behaved as if they were a different person; and that they found letters and drawings which were conspicuously their own productions but bore a different signature; and, most importantly, that they had no recollection of these acts. One could intuitively deduce that they would begin to lose confidence in the validity of their experience. At the very least, they would call into question their criteria for distinguishing reality from fantasy. Such existential insecurity would seriously undermine the development of an ego, a central regulator, whose role is the constant surveillance of all the person's experience, and the arbiter of what is real and what is imagined. The way would now be paved for some substitute to coordinate one's mental life, a kind of mental prosthesis, which would not only be trusted but on which one would place total reliance. The hypnotist could embody just such a surrogate ego.

What is being suggested is that there may be an, as yet unidentified, set of characteristics which predisposes individuals to be highly hypnotisable and/or multiple personalities.

Although he makes no explicit reference to multiple personality, Spiegel (1974) seems to be thinking along the same lines when he identifies the "Grade 5 Syndrome." The term derives from high scorers on a 0–5 hypnotisability range, as measured by the Hypnotic Induction Profile (HIP). It is Spiegel's experience that high scorers are not only highly hypnotisable but that "under duress the grade 5 becomes the so-called hysterical patient."

Such individuals represent no more than 10% of the population and exhibit a distinctive constellation of 10 behavioural and personality attributes.

Firstly, they show a high eye-roll (ER). This ER is constant and is relatively unaffected by practice which leads Spiegel to propose either genetic basis or acquisition during an early imprinting phase.

Second, they have "an intense, beguilingly innocent expectation of support from others ... [an] incredibly demanding faith ... a lack of cynicism. Whatever the difficulties of their therapy, they retain faith, hope, trust, and the conviction that therapy is 'good' for them." This, Spiegel calls their posture of trust.

Thirdly, deriving from their trust is a "willingness to replace, if necessary, old premises and beliefs with new ones, without the usual cognitive screenings and scrutinisings" of those who score low on the HIP. This receptivity, this suspension of critical judgement, makes them more than usually prone to wreak changes in the system of beliefs and metaphors (what Spiegel terms, the metaphor-mix) through which they construe their worlds.

Fourthly, Spiegel believes that grade 5s have highly developed empathic abilities which make them prone to affiliate with new events. He cites the case of Dorothy who "on seeing a friend's dog sick with nausea... promptly became nauseated herself; such was her receptiveness to others."

Fifth is an ability to focus almost exclusively on the present, a relatively telescoped time sense. The fact that grade 5s are capable of age regression is only an apparent paradox since the age to which they regress then becomes their present. Thus unlike lower HIP scorers, they are not just receiving fragmental impressions which are seen against the backcloth of the ever present now. Whereas the low scorers will report that they are recalling past events, grade 5s will vividly re-experience them and they will be isolated from current decision making.

Sixthly, they will reveal a tolerance for logical inconsistencies, the trance logic described by Orne (1959). Spiegel points out that such tolerance of contradiction can be very comfortable. To illustrate he uses the example of "army logic" when we are told that "in order to secure a village we have to destroy it ... for most, of us, of course, it is very difficult to make peace with that kind of 'logic' because it violates so many other premises as well as our ordinary means of dealing with them."

A timely digression is to note the peculiar difficulty in feeling comfortable with the notion of multiple personality because it seems to use just such logical inconsistency. One person, one personality, is the norm and to moot the possibility of a single psyche composed of discrete "selves" seems to violate not just experience but also deeply instantiated rules about what is, and what is not, logically possible. What must not be forgotten is that the individual employing "trance logic" is making a mistake! No matter how comforting it might be to accept passively apparent contradictions, this does not permit dismantling the laws of logic. Nor does it change objective reality. The "sound of one hand clapping", or the perception of three-sided squares, are not elevated beyond the level of non-sense because they are the reported experiences of devout religious mystics. If a village is under enemy occupation, then its destruction becomes a rational (albeit morally questionable) tactic in securing it. Ignorance of covert organising principles does not mean they do not exist and the blithe tolerance of inconsistency is a luxury the scientist cannot afford.

The seventh hallmark of the grade 5s is their excellent rote and eidetic memory and their ability for total recall which enhances their ability to regress under hypnosis.

The eighth defining attribute is their intense capacity for concentration and concurrent dissociation. Spiegel's examples are writers and painters who describe their artistic productions as if they "created themselves." For instance, he quotes a novelist as saying, "That character fascinates me; it's as if I didn't write him; he created himself – and I kept getting more and more amazed at what he was doing as we went along in the story." Spiegel goes on to state, "This intense concentration is what makes the creator able to be both with his creation and alongside it at the same time; to relate to that concentration in a guided, disciplined, yet dissociated way. This is the critical feature that emphasises the perceptual alteration common to all hypnosis; the observed motor phenomena are secondary to the perceptual shift."

In a footnote, Spiegel comments on the unsuitability of "hypnosis" as a term given etymology in the Greek word meaning "sleep". He wonders whether a suitable replacement might not be a phrase which captured the notion of parallel streams of consciousness such as "multiple awareness," or "dual perception." Comparison with "multiple personality" is inescapable.

Penultimately, Spiegel refers to a fixed personality core, underlying the surface changeability, and receptivity of grade 5s, which is especially resistant to change or therapeutic intervention. One of his illustrations was a woman with hysterical seizures. Although she learned that her seizures could be brought under hypnotic control "she insisted on retaining a certain cycle of response. She would predictably take about a minute to come out of the seizure after having been signalled to do so. This minute gradually was reduced, but she still insisted on holding on to a little hard-core refractory period."

Finally, Spiegel notes role confusion with a reactive sense of inferiority which he believes derives from this paradox between the hard-core dynamism and "chameleon-like malleable overlay". He suggests that embarrassment, as well as inferiority feelings, may accompany achievement because individuals will feel only minimally responsible for their successes. Spiegel refers to an anatomy student who felt his exam success was tantamount to cheating since all he had done was to "copy" from his vivid eidetic images. Since the memorising ability of grade 5s is typically of a mechanistic, rote nature, with little real understanding or integration of knowledge, Spiegel sees a realistic basis for such unease.

Spiegel's delineation of the grade 5 syndrome is a fascinating and insightful account of a finite complex of traits which warrants more detailed quantitative analysis. Even as it stands, it provides a rich hypothetical framework for those investigators who would prefer to seek a premorbid basis for both hypnotisability and multiple personality rather than trying, exclusively, to explain either one in terms of the other.

The following chapter examines a different attempt to bring these two phenomena under a conceptually distinct rubric, namely that of role theory.

CHAPTER 7

A Social Perspective

Inevitably, the preceding discussion of multiple personality has included passim reference to a variety of theoretical perspectives. These range from psychodynamic and object-relations approaches on the one hand to physiological accounts on the other. What they have in common is an implicit acknowledgement that multiple personality is somehow a "real" phenomenon with a discrete and distinctive existence. They also share an emphasis on explanations which locate the source of the behaviour within the individual. Thus we have become familiar with notions such as splitting, and dissociated ego-states with their more-or-less permeable boundaries. Multiple personality patients have also been conceptualised as premorbidly at risk owing to "psychic readiness" or proneness to the abuse of self-hypnosis. In Chapter 5, for example, I wrote about several, slightly differing attempts to identify multiple personalities with hemispheric differences. Here, however, I am concerned to present an approach which sharply contrasts with all such "individualistic" accounts and which has already been briefly referred to in earlier chapters. Such an approach is conspicuously rooted in the paradigm of social psychology and relatedly of sociology.

One way of describing the social psychological enterprise to the layman, or beginning student, is to talk in terms of traditional foci of social psychological research. Thus one might make reference to group dynamics; leadership and conformity; non-verbal communication and social attraction; or attitude formation and change. However, modern introductory texts will quickly point out that the essence of social psychology lies more in its basic ideology than in its content. What is distinctive about the social psychological (and, for that matter, the sociological) enterprise is its epistemology rather than its subject matter.

Unlike "individual" psychologists, exemplified by personality theorists and intelligence testers, social psychologists eschew explanations in terms of intra-individual variables in favour of those which stress inter-individual processes. At the micro level this means an emphasis on the relationships between individuals, and between individuals and the diverse, relatively small, groups of which they are a member or which they aspire to join. At a more macro level of explanation, there is a concern with the impact of society and culture on behaviour. It is overly simplistic to see such an approach as merely complementary to one that prefers to lay stress on the individual, say, in terms of "traits" or neurotransmitters. Such an approach can lie starkly at variance with those that favour explanation in terms of idiodynamics, or of stable and enduring individual differences.

At root, the social psychologist (and sociologist) are arguing that nurture counts for rather more than nature, and that there is a plasticity to human behaviour which allows for radical change. It is hardly surprising, therefore, that such an epistemolgial difference should have been politicised, with the advocates of human potentiality for constant change being construed as more left wing than those who read our destiny in our genes or, at least, our biological constitution. However, I leave it to my sociological colleagues to uncover scientific mileage in such conceptualisations.

It is also the hallmark of socially couched theorising to focus on present rather than on past influences on behaviour. Their concern, accordingly, is with current socio-economic forces, with the prevailing social consciousness. Such a contemporaneous approach does not mean that the social psychologist does not believe that, for example, our childhood has no bearing on adult behaviour. What it does do is to argue that what is important are our current cognitive representations of our history and the history of our reference groups together with the contemporaneous demands of the here-and-now social setting.

In this way, most contemporary social psychologists also adopt a cognitive, phenomenological standpoint. We shall see shortly, however, that even pre-eminent social psychologists are sometimes curiously incurious about investigating the mental worlds of their experimental subjects. For, experimental subjects are also experiential subjects.

Multiple personality patients are extraordinarily similar to each other. If for no other reason, this would make the presentation of more than a sample of case history extracts both tedious and redundant. Not only do they commonly have a childhood history of psychological and/or physical abuse but their alter egos, no matter how many, tend to fall into three broadly defined groups. There are those that are extravert, sexually self-conscious, mischievous and, at the extreme, aggressive and promiscuous. In contrast, there are the introverted personae, sexually and socially inhibited, and, it would seem, normally the initially presenting host personality. Thirdly, there are the stable "hidden observers", dare one say "happy mediums", like Eve's Jane and Sybil's Vicky, who are reported as both intervening to avert disaster and as allying with the therapist to achieve integration. These personalities tend to be the favourites with their therapists, and tend to "come out" more and more often as therapy progresses.

The very sameness of the presentations, it might be argued, is grist to the mill of those who would have us believe that multiple personality is a real clinical entity. There are, however, alternative explanations of such uniformity, deriving from more social psychological platforms.

The social psychologist argues that much of our behaviour can be explained in terms of the roles that we are enacting at any particular time. Role Theory is predicated on the notion that we are all members of groups, and that it is our perception of the dynamics of these groups that generates the roles that we enact. Such groups may be as small as two, as common as the family, or as all-embracing as the larger society in which we live.

There is a comforting familiarity about the concept of "role" given that a moment's introspection reveals to us all that we occupy an enormous diversity of roles in daily life, and that our behaviour is continually a product of the role we happen to be occupying at any particular moment.

As I sit and write this monograph I occupy the role of psychological researcher and essayist using a prosaic style which would sound distinctly odd were I to employ it in conversation at my local pub. The telephone rings and I find myself speaking to my mother, who asks how I am coping with the cold weather. Am I wearing warm clothes and "looking after myself"? In the role of child, I not only reassure her but confess to a minor stomach upset which I have never mentioned to my children who I feel would be unduly worried by their Daddy's ailment. The doorbell rings and I am engaged in a scenario with a policeman informing me that the tax disc on my car, parked outside, is out of date. Will I see to its renewal, promptly? With all deference I assure him of my good intent, feeling sincerely anxious during our formal encounter. Within minutes of returning to my monograph a student from college telephones to seek advice about where to go next in their essay assignment and with all the assurance of a college lecturer I proffer directive advice. Different roles, different experience and behaviour, all within the space of a few minutes. The enactment of social roles is not always such a straightforward successive affair since different roles often run parallel to each other. Sometimes such role parallelism may be harmonious as when the schoolteacher helps their child with homework. Sometimes role conflict can be generated as when the schoolteacher discovers that their child has been cheating during an examination.

Seemingly, role theory is an easy approach to grasp. So accessible, indeed, that one might question whether such a mundane perspective warranted the nomenclature of a "theory". However, "theory" or no, such an approach has profound implications and creates pitfalls for the unwary. Conceptualising human behaviour as role enactments can be misunderstood as suggesting that we are all permanently leading a life of self-conscious pretence. It might seem that a role-theory account of mental illness, for example, could reduce to an argument that all psychiatric patients are malingerers. Nothing could be further from the intent. For role-theory to have anything important to say it is essential that we bear in mind that roles are not only situational but that they have phenomenological as well as behavioural dimensions. Whilst writing my monograph, talking to my mother, my children, a policeman or my student there will be conspicuous differences in my behaviour. For example, my posture and tone of voice, even my accent may alter. However, I not only behave differently, I feel differently. I reconstrue my world. My self-concept undergoes radical alterations but it is unlikely that I will be aware of these myriad metamorphoses.

Role-taking is not an all-or-none affair. Instead we become more or less absorbed in our everyday dramas just as professional actors, during the long run of a play, will find themselves more "lost" in their role on some occasions than others. Actors report that they sometimes cry "real" tears, or experience "genuine" hatred or affection toward other player when on stage. To the extent that we are role-involved we lose self-consciousness. The more self-aware we become the more does our behaviour represent pretence, deception or malingering. Commonly acute self-awareness can positively hamper effective performance. We are all used to behaving rather clumsily during the most well-practised skills when under the eye of a prominent observer. Masters and Johnson (1970) have pointed out how sexual performance can be impaired when partners adopt a "spectator role". Therapy comprises focusing on bodily sensations whilst being massaged by one's partner and abandoning oneself unself-consciously to the experience of sexuality.

Unself-conscious role- playing and the deliberate charade are the opposite poles of a continuum, at some point along which a qualitative change takes place in the same way that water metamorphoses, by degree, into ice or steam. The complexity of human behaviour, however, does not allow social scientists anything like the precision of chemists and physicists in earmarking such points of transition.

Congdon, Hain and Stevenson (1961) present the case of a 23- year-old housewife whose primary personality was known as Betty. They suggest that she illustrates the transition between an imaginary playmate, simple role-playing and dual personality.

On admission she presented with hysterical convulsions and severe depression. During psychotherapy she referred to an imaginary childhood playmate called Elizabeth and, some 2 months later suddenly "sat bolt upright in her chair, at the same time assuming a more relaxed and friendly demeanour, and said to the therapist: 'I think it's about time I started telling you about me.'" Elizabeth had apparently taken over, and switching between the two personalities continued for 4 months.

Betty was tense, stiff and formal. She was introverted and complained of headaches, abdominal cramps, dysmennorrhoea and frequent fainting. Elizabeth, on the other hand, was extraverted and humorous, spoke in a higher pitch, and was physically healthy. She knew of Betty's existence but denied that she (Elizabeth) was married. Betty was amnesic for Elizabeth's behaviour and experience. Approximately fifty transitions occurred, taking 10 seconds or so each time, without hypnosis, at the therapist's bidding.

The Rorschach, Hutt Sentence Completion Test, Orzeck Self Scale and Word Association Test were presented to both personalities. The authors report that the Rorschachs were similar in that both showed compulsive thought processes, an inability to be objective and perceptions were easily influenced by emotions. Betty evidenced more fantasy and less emotional lability than Elizabeth who, in turn, was less socially conforming and impulsively hedonistic.

On the Sentence Completion Test, Betty was more childlike and rule-bound, fearful and derogated men. Elizabeth was rebellious, liked men, and said she feared nothing.

Both showed similar word-associations save for sexual topics which provoked negative associations from Betty in contrast to more hedonistic or neutral responses from Elizabeth.

The Orzeck Self-Scale, which the authors baldly state is "more open to conscious control and evaluation than any of the foregoing psychological tests" provoked 43 "maladjusted" responses from Betty as compared with only 4 such responses from Elizabeth, suggesting that Elizabeth was the more psychologically healthy of the two personalities. The summary was, that over all the tests, the personalities differed only in areas charged with anxiety.

Betty's history was the familiar one of loss and abuse. Her father committed suicide when she was 4 and parenting was largely undertaken by a tyrannical grandmother who communicated fear and disgust toward sex. When she was 5 Betty was sexually assaulted by a neighbour and, at age 7, Betty reported that Elizabeth was created as an imaginary companion who was maintained through high school. Betty would deliberately play the role of Elizabeth when she went to the few parties she was allowed to attend. In this role she said that she was able to relax and enjoy herself more.

At 19 she married her only suitor who turned out to be brutal and sexually deviant. Congdon et al., apropos of the first spontaneous transition, write that once "when her husband behaved in a particularly cruel manner, the patient suddenly became unusually aggressive and chased him from the home. She (Betty) had amnesia for this episode." The evidence for this is based on retrospective accounts of relatives (presumably biased against the husband) which Congdon "pieced together". His interpretation is that Elizabeth had come out to protect Betty and was to remain "out" for 6 months during which she had an affair.

Her husband divorced her for adultery, and it seems that the stress of the divorce combined with a return to her grandmother's home, precipitated Betty's hysterical convulsions and hospital admission.

During the 4 months of therapy Elizabeth worked as an ally of the therapist, filling in Betty's history where she was amnesic for Elizabeth's actions. Gradually, Betty became aware of Elizabeth's presence which Congdon et al. saw as resembling the earlier period of conscious role-playing. Finally, Elizabeth ceased to emerge and Betty, with full recall for all she had done as Elizabeth, left her grandmother's home and took a job in another town.

In their discussion, the authors argue, acknowledging Taylor and Martin (1944), that habitual roles can become "hardened" into secondary personalities. Such a transition can be the product of differential reinforcement by the therapist or family members, an artefact of hypnosis, or the prolonged use of an imaginary playmate where conscious role-playing leads to favourable outcomes. Given Betty's repressive upbringing, they argue that the transition to conscious role-playing in adolescence was a natural development. They go on to say that the crucial feature for a diagnosis of multiple personality is the presence of amnesia, putatively serving an adaptive function, where dissociation becomes consolidated into repression.

Was Betty just an actress? Congdon et al. insist that she would have needed extraordinary skill if this were the case, and the consistency of her performance and its existence prior to therapy impressed them she was genuine. However, it has already been argued that the degree of skill required is vastly overrated, and it is a harsh truth that human beings devote much of their lives to consistent and utterly convincing deceptions. The crime columns of the daily press are replete with stories of villains who have lived normal lives as loving spouses and parents. They hold down jobs as respected members of the community, sometimes as members of youth movements and law enforcement agencies. Should one be too surprised? Such occupations not only provide "cover". They also afford special opportunities to be near young prey or to subvert the course of justice. However, it is eventually revealed that such "pillars of the community" have spent years as thieves, sexual deviants, rapists or even murderers, to the astonishment of all their close acquaintances.

To paraphrase Sarbin (Sarbin and Anderson, 1967), successful role-enactment depends on:

1. Role expectations (how one expects to behave in a given situation).
2. Role perceptions (how one interprets the demand characteristics of the situation, one's "stage directions").
3. Role relevant skills (e.g. a vivid imagination).
4. Self-role congruence (how far one's conception of the role to be played is in tune or at odds with one's current self-concept).
5. Sensitivity to role demands (e.g. awareness that non-compliance may offend other actors in the scenario).

One might add to this list, the availability of appropriate role models.

In this context it is pertinent to look at the findings of two social psychological experiments of Nicholas Spanos, Professor of Psychology at Ottawa's Carleton University.

Spanos et al. (1985) argue that multiple personality patients are far from being the passive victims of internal, unconscious processes. Rather, they are purposeful participants in acting out the role of such patients "using available information to create a social impression that is congruent with their perception of situational demands and with the interpersonal goals they are attempting to achieve." Assisting in the scenario are their therapists who not only provide encouragement, information and "stage direction" in impression management but who, perhaps most important, provide "official validation" for the different identities enacted, especially when one personality is enlisted as a therapeutic ally.

Similarly, "hypnotic procedures are conceptualised as rituals that, in the context of psychotherapy may serve to legitimate the transition from manifestations of one identity to manifestations of another." Spanos notes that the experiments of Kampman (1976) and Watkins and Watkins (1980) show how highly hypnotisable college students will report, via hypnotic suggestion, the presence of multiple inner selves.

Information (stage directions) about such role enactment is also widely available, especially in the United States' culture. Key examples are the books and films about

Eve and Sybil together with the more recent film, *Dressed To Kill*, where a male psychoanalyst (no less) adopts a murderous, female alter-ego who attacks females who arouse him sexually. The widely publicised cases of Milligan and Bianchi, and the newsletter, *Speaking For Ourselves* , referred to in the first chapter, are further readily available sources for multiple personality life-scripts. (One is indebted to Goffman (1969) whose brilliant dramaturgical analysis of social behaviour introduced such terminolgy as "impression management" and "scripts" into the technical vocabulary of social psychology. Perhaps because Goffman is a sociologist rather than a psychologist, he has sometimes been unduly acknowledged in the psychological literature.)

Spanos goes on to reiterate the sentiments of Thigpen and Cleckley (1984), that the role of multiple personality is relatively attractive, "portraying the protagonist as a person with a dramatic set of symptoms who overcomes numerous obstacles and eventually gains dignity, esteem, and much sympathetic attention from significant, high-status others." Within one week of this writer's public announcement of his intention to write this book, a young woman presented herself, together with a photographic portfolio, claiming to be suffering from multiple personality. She was a model who thought that the variety of parts she played to the camera indicated such a condition. Not only may the role seem attractive but it has already been observed that it can provide an apologia for otherwise intolerable behaviour.

Spanos is unimpressed by "state theorists". He has this to say about EEG and visual-evoked response studies:

> These results [Braun, 1983; Larmore, Ludwig and Cain, 1977; Ludwig et al., 1972] are far from conclusive. For instance, Lamore, Ludwig and Cain reported VER differences between the four personality enactments of a single multiple, and concluded that it was 'as if four different people had been tested '(p. 40). However, their data indicate as much variability within as between the various personality enactments. Moreover, Ludwig, Brandsma, Wilbur, Benfeldt and Jameson (1972) and Coons, Milstein and Marley (1982) found no VER differences between multiples. [Both sets of researchers] reported EEG differences between the personality enactments of their patients. It is important, however, that Coons, Milstein and Marley also found that a non-patient control who simulated different personalities produced even more marked between-personality EEG differences than did the actual patients.

From the social-learning perspective, Spanos cites Kohlenberg's (1973) study of a patient diagnosed as having three personalities. After baseline rates for the occurrence of personality-specific behaviours had been established, behaviours specific to one persona were selectively reinforced and showed a dramatic increase in frequency.

The springboard for the experiment of Spanos et al. was the Bianchi case, presented in Chapter 2. Forty eight undergraduate subjects (24 male, 24 female) volunteered to role-play an accused murderer named Harry or Betty. They were told nothing about the multiple personality syndrome. Eight men and eight women were randomly assigned to one of three experimental conditions. These were three interview treatments varying in the degree to which they cued for manifesting multiple personality.

In the first condition, following almost verbatim the treatment of Bianchi, subjects were asked, "Part, are you the same thing as Harry (Betty) or are you different?" In the second condition, subjects were told that personality was complex but that hypnosis could get behind the "wall" that hid inner thoughts and feelings from awareness. They were also told that during hypnosis the hypnotists would be able to talk with a different part of them. In the third, non-hypnotic, control condition, subjects were told merely that personality was complex and included walled-off thoughts and feelings.

Spanos also administered twice a five-item sentence completion and a semantic differential test to all subjects (in each of their roles, where a second personality was enacted). The sentence completion test dealt with self, mother, least liked aspect of self, sexual thoughts and anger. The semantic differential employed the same concepts used by Osgood and Luria (1957) to evaluate Eve's "three selves".

Subjects were told that they were to play the role of accused multiple murderer whose defence lawyer had entered a not guilty plea. They would be interviewed by a "psychiatrist" who might use hypnosis in which case they were also to role-play being hypnotised. They were also informed that it was normal procedure with such court referrals to videotape the sessions.

After the opening remarks by the "psychiatrist" (concerning the complexity of personality etc.) subjects were asked:

1. Who are you?
2. Tell me about yourself?
3. Do you have a name I can call you by?
4. Tell me about yourself (using name used by subject in response to Q.3), what do you do?

Responses were rated by judges who were blind to subjects's treatment groups. Inter-rater agreement ranged from 92% to 100%.

The results were in the direction Spanos predicted: 81% of subjects in the Bianchi treatment, and 31% of subjects in the hidden-part treatment adopted a name other then Harry or Betty. Of those subjects who adopted a different name 70% also referred to two different identities. For example, one said , "I'm sort of like Harry's friend, 'cause Harry didn't have many friends when he was little." Another said, "I've always been with Betty since I can remember. She doesn't know I'm here, but I know I'm here."

63% of subjects in both hypnotic treatments also displayed spontaneous amnesia. No control subjects used another name or portrayed amnesia.

Almost all subjects initially denied guilt but, following treatment administration, subjects in the two hypnotic conditions were significantly more likely to admit guilt (P< .01).

Spanos then compared the two sets of test results of the 11 subjects who used a second name and portrayed amnesia ("multiples") with the 23 "nonmultiples" who displayed neither. Multiples wrote significantly more sentences on the sentence completion task (P < .001). Difference scores on the semantic differential were analysed with a 211 split-plot analysis of variance (ANOVA) with one between-subjects factor (multiple personality/no multiple personality) and one within-subjects factor (11 constructs). The main effect for groups indicated that multiples obtained significantly higher difference scores than non-multiples (P < .001). Nonmultiples also took significantly less time to read the test instructions on the second administration (P < .001).

In his subsequent discussion Spanos makes four points. First, he notes that only subjects in the hypnotic conditions used another name, reported two different identities, and also reported amnesia, for which they were not cued. Does this not indicate the crucial role of the situational demands on subjects' performance? Second, is the fact that all but one of the multiples admitted guilt on the second administration whilst all nonmultiples who had initially denied guilt continued to do so. Does this not suggest that multiples were prepared to admit guilt because the existence of another self had now been legitimised; another self to whom all blame could be apportioned? Nonmultiples, having no such legitimised scapegoat, could but maintain their innocence. Third, Spanos challenges Watkins' (1984) assertion that naive individuals could not fake multiple personality. Spanos writes, "our findings indicate rather clearly that when given the appropriate inducements, enacting the multiple personality role is a relatively easy task." He goes on to point out that the whole "script" does not have to be written. A large degree of improvisation takes place once some basic rules have been established. Let us not underestimate human inventiveness. In this way, one will encounter, for example, references to oneself in the third person, a disavowal of responsibility for the activities of the "other" even to the extent of reporting amnesia, together with different responses to the same psychological tests.

Finally, Spanos makes the important point that multiples typically portray sharply contrasting alter-egos. For some reason, we have seen constantly that this has led commentators to be all the more impressed with their patients' presentations. Spanos argues, quite simply, that such a sharp contrast is surely in the interests of "cognitive economy." (I have argued earlier that it is demonstrably more easy to play sharply contrasting roles than it is to offer one's audience subtle nuances of change in personal identity. It is the latter that requires the skills of an accomplished actor.) Also, how much easier it must be to remember all the idiosyncracies of Personality A, rather than Personality B, where A and B are stereotypical opposites. Is this not a more economical explanation of the observed consistency in the behaviour of an alternate personality?

Does the elegantly designed research of Spanos allow us to subsume multiple personality syndrome under the head of role-play, of a subspecies of social learning? Or is the research too artificial, too "laboratory-bound"? Does it lack ecological validity?

The accused criminal can have much to gain from an insanity plea. As much as their life. Does this mean that forensic psychiatric investigations create unique demands or provide unique cues? Spanos argues that patients in psychotherapy are victim to a similar degree of social constraint. They, too, are engaged in social interactions with high-status experts who have to be taken seriously. Additionally, they are frequently unhappy, insecure and of low self-esteem. The situation is rife for them to seek ways of winning their therapist's approval, interest and concern. Paraphrasing Sutcliffe and Jones (1962), Spanos says that "under these circumstances, mutual shaping between therapists "on the lookout" for signs of multiple personality and clients involved in conveying an appropriate impression, may lead to enactments of multiple personality that confirm the initial suspicions of the therapist and that, in turn, lead the therapist to encourage and to validate more elaborate displays of the disorder ...(given that) clinicians vary quite dramatically in the extent to which they deem it appropriate to encourage and legitimate enactments of multiple identity it is little wonder ...that some therapists are much more likely than others to "discover" cases of multiple personality, or that the recent upsurge in the number of such patients parallels increased interest in the disorder and increased sensitivity ot signs that call for interview procedures like those used with Bianchi."

Spanos interprets the amnesia of his subjects as a "strategic enactment" whereby memory processes are controlled to guide recall (and failure to recall) in response to the situational demands of an hypnotic scenario (e.g. Spanos, Radtke, and Bertrand, 1984).

In the same fashion, Spanos interprets patients' "fusion of dissociated identities" as but one more set of responses when the interaction between therapist and patient has been "(redefined) as one in which displays of 'cross personality' remembering are now considered role appropriate."

He is at pains to stress that his social psychological perspective does not exclude the possibility of predisposing personal attributes and cognitive styles such as a vivid imagination, rich fantasy life or hypnotic susceptibility. However, it should be noted that Spanos's subjects also completed the Carleton University Responsiveness to Suggestion Scale (CURSS) but a chi-square analysis did not differentiate between multiples (different name plus amnesia) and nonmultiples. He adds, "when interpreting these results it is important to keep in mind that subjects were instructed to role play a defendant undergoing hypnosis. They were not instructed to, themselves, become 'hypnotised'." It is not at all clear, however, what such a distinction might mean to a role theorist.

Finally, Spanos refers to investigators such as Orne, Dinges and Orne (1984) who state that the diagnosis of multiple personality requires evidence of the pretherapy existence of multiple personalities. Apart from the problem that such evidence is typically based on reports of the patients themselves during therapy, or upon the retrospective and, often ambiguous, accounts of relatives and friends, Spanos has this to say: "it is not clear that cases involving evidence of pretherapy multiple identity enactment should be considered somehow more genuine than are those in which the relevant self-conceptions and other role components were learned and first enacted in the therapist's office."

Despite the elegance and rigour of the experiment of Spanos et al. some may find the results an unconvincing refutation of the "state theory" approach to multiple personality given that his paradigm was procedure with a criminal who was eventually exposed as faking the syndrome.

There is the additional problem that Spanos' enquiries stopped short of asking his subjects how they "felt" when acting out their roles as defendant, as multiple personality patient, and as hypnotised. The state theorist will surely want to argue for a difference in subjective experience between the "genuine" defendant, or multiple personality patient, or hypnotised subject, and the actor. Given the absence of any objective indices of being a multiple personality or of being hypnotised (it is salutary to recall that even Milton Erikson could not distinguish between "simulators" and "reals") is one not obliged to seek differences in reported subjective experience?

In this context, I remember attending my first hypnosis workshop. We (a collection of medical doctors, dentists and psychologists) had been divided into small groups each led by an experienced hypnotist. In my group, a general practitioner had volunteered to be a subject for the hypotist who explained that he was going to put the doctor into a light trance (sic) and then induce a feeling of lightness in the doctor's arm so that it would levitate. The doctor closed his eyes, was duly hypnotised and, after what seemed a tediously long period of suggestion, his limb slowly raised from the arm of the chair and remained suspended in the air. The hypnotist, with what seemed like a sigh of relief, then suggested to the doctor that he would be unable to lower his arm. To my own naive wonderment the doctor then seemed to struggle vainly to lower his arm. Finally, the hypnotist told the doctor that it was now all right to lower his arm and the doctor duly complied. At this point the group broke up for a coffee break and I eagerly sought out the doctor and expressed some incredulity at what I had witnessed. He smiled benignly and confessed something like the following (as soon as he had finished his account I made a note of what he confided, as near verbatim as possible): "I can sympathise with your scepticism because that's just how I felt when I volunteered. In fact, when Dr Gibson (the psychologist/hypnotist, and Chair of the British Society of Clinical and Experimental Hypnosis) first began suggesting that my arm was getting lighter and lighter I felt nothing of the kind. It started to get a bit embarrassing and I felt as if I was making him look a bit of a fool. He seemed such a nice chap that I decided, a bit irresponsibly perhaps, to pretend that it really was floating up in the air. So I slowly raised it and kept it there while I heard him tell the group I would be unable to lower it. By now my arm was beginning to ache and I was in something of a quandary. My discomfort wasn't going to allow me to keep my arm up for much longer but I wanted to keep up my pretence. I then decided that enough was enough! I shouldn't have embarked on such a charade in the first place. I would lower my arm and admit my deception to the group. But I couldn't! I really tried to lower my arm but it seemed to have an existence of its own. And, what I found really remarkable was that the discomfort had gone. I think I could have kept it up there for ages. Even when it came down it seemed to be doing it by itself."

What is one to make of such an introspective account? Is it sufficient evidence of a meaningful distinction between "real states" and role-playing? I doubt that the social psychologist would find it too persuasive. The account could be reconstrued as differences in degree of self-awareness with a concomitantly increased absorbtion in one's role. The professional actor who feigns sadness at Monday's performance, and cries real tears on Tuesday's stage, is none the less acting on both occasions. He knows on both nights that he is not really a Moorish prince who has murdered his wife.

After (Frank, 1973), Spanos et al. (1986), in their more recent paper, summarise their position on multiple personality: "the biographical accounts proffered by psychotherapy patients reflect a complex interweaving of veridically recalled past experience and much retrospective distortion and elaboration that is organised in terms of patients' current concerns and implicit theories of psychopathology." They add, "adopting the role of a multiple usually requires that patients construct a past history that is consistent with their self-presentation as possessing multiple identities."

The experiment of Spanos et al. (1986) was typically elegant and complex. In part it replicated their 1984 study but it also looked at age regression since this technique is commonly used to allow patients and therapists "access" to secondary personalities. Such personalities are most often reported as emerging before age 10, and different personalities may provide differing evaluations of relationships with parents. Secondary personalities are also typically described as serving specific functions. As well as examining these ideas, Spanos et al. anticipated that role-playing subjects would present their alter-egos as more psychopathological than their primary identity. (This may seem counter-intuitive, since secondary personalities are typically described as being better adjusted. These seem to be the "copers", dealing with stressful encounters, intervening in suicide attempts and even being employed as therapeutic aides. In the present context, however, it should be recalled that Allison (1984) and Watkins (1984) reported that Bianchi's Rorschach and CPI responses were more psychopathological when tested as Steve rather than as Ken, the primary personality.)

Eighty subjects (40 male and 40 female) took part in a three-session experiment where they were asked to role play an accused murderer. In session one, they were interviewed about their relationship with the "victim" and about their childhood. They also completed the schizophrenia and psychopathic deviate scales of the MMPI and a questionnaire concerning their perception of their parents, as well as the sentence completion test and semantic differential employed in the earlier (Spanos et al.,1984) study. In session two, half the subjects (20 male and 20 female, randomly assigned) were given the Bianchi hypnotic interview treatment together with instructions for age regression. The remaining, non-hypnotic control, subjects were simply asked to close their eyes, think back to particular ages and recall the significant events of that period. In the third session, subjects were reinterviewed and again completed the test battery. Where subjects had manifested a different identity in the second session, this personality was "called forth" to complete the procedures. Otherwise subjects were asked to continue role playing accused murderer.

A different identity was reported by 60% of Bianchi treatment subjects (χ^2 (1)=39.29, P< .001); 80% of Bianchi treatment subjects also spontaneously reported amnesia. No controls reported either phenomenon. Only two control and one Bianchi treatment subject initially admitted guilt. However, following the treatment manipulation, 10 of the Bianchi subjects admitted guilt whereas no controls changed their plea ($\chi^2(1)$=10.79, P<001).

66% of the role-playing multiples reported that their secondary personalities performed specific functions, e.g. acting as "friend" or handling strong emotions.

Reported ages of the first emergence of secondary personalities ranged from birth to 20 years (M=6.58, SD=5.11) with 81% reporting emergence before age 10. All multiples referred to their secondary personalities in the third person.

A one-way ANOVA revealed that multiples demonstrated more differences in their relationships with others across the two interviews (F(1,54)=34.82, P< .001). For example, one subject while role playing Harry said his relationships with women were "pretty good" but in his secondary personality said, "I don't relate to them ... I let Harry do all that. But if they get him angry, I will come out."

After "regression" to the earliest age they had indicated, multiples provided more negative descriptions than did nonmultiple controls (F(1,45)=4.21, P< .05).

Multiples also showed more differences across the two sentence completion tasks (F(1,55)=54.75, P< .001). For example, one subject, as Betty, wrote "My father is a teacher" but in her secondary personality, wrote "My father is mean."

The semantic differential responses were subjected to separate 22 ANOVAS on each concept with Multiple Personality/No Multiple Personality as a between-subjects factor and Testings1/2 as a within-subjects factor. These ANOVAS yielded significant interactions for eight of the ten concepts. There was no difference between multiples and nonmultiples on baseline testing, nor did nonmultiples significantly change their ratings over the two testings. Multiples, however, were significantly more likely to give more negative ratings to concepts on the second testing.

Multiples also rated themselves as significantly less close to their parents on the second testing whereas nonmultiples showed no such difference in "parental distance" over the two testings. There was no difference on baseline testing between multiples and nonmultiple controls.

The MMPI scales were subjected to a 22 (Multiple/Nonmultiple Testings 1/2) mixed ANOVA and yielded significant interactions (Sc, F(1,55)=10.64, P< .01, Pd, F(1,55=9.22, P< .01). Thus on the second testing, multiples described their secondary personalities as more psychopathological than their primary personality. There were no baseline differences between multiples and nonmultiples, nor did nonmultiple controls show any significant change in MMPI responses over the two testings.

Thus, Spanos et al. replicated and extended their earlier findings that interview treatments that encourage and legitimise role-playing can produce many of the phenomena of multiple personality. These include the adoption of a differently named identity, use of the third person in self-reference, spontaneously reported amnesia, eventual admission of guilt, consistent differences in response on psychological tests and differences in historical accounts of childhood relationships and of current relationships to others.

In their discussion of these results, Spanos et al. (1986) point to a large body of research (e.g. Braginsky and Braginsky (1967); Berglas and Jones, 1978; Jones and Berglas, 1978; Snyder and Smith, 1982; Smith et al., 1983; DeGree and Snyder, 1985) which demonstrates that individuals tend to attribute past difficulties and anticipated failures to alleged psychopathology. Relatedly, professionals are ideologically predisposed to explain current transgressions in terms of "damaging" childhood experience. The stage is set for collusion in the construction of life histories which somehow construe, and even condone, present psychopathology as the outcome of forces to which the multiple personality patient is a passive victim. Biographies will be provided where parents are described as distant and rejecting, secondary personalties began to emerge during childhood and these personalties had specific functions, for example, to fend off aggressors or handle difficult affects. This is not to say that such interview situations are the only or necessary circumstances which will generate such role playing.

It is important to note the conclusion of Spanos et al. that multiple personality patients are not generally to be regarded as engaged in conscious deception. An equally important rider, however, is that the absence of any objective indices of this putative disorder means that it can be feigned and one needs to be especially aware of this possibility when examining patients accused of criminal activities.

Neither this monograph nor the perspective of social psychology are simply concerned with the issue of "real" versus "fake" multiple personality patients. The concern is more with the issues of, under what circumstances are individuals likely to be so labelled and what are the implications of such labelling? Therapists, family and friends are all likely to be involved in legitimising the adoption of such roles. If multiple personality patients are victim to anything, it is to their own role enactments and the reinforcement of their therapists. Thus all players in the scenario come sincerely to believe in whole hosts of alternate personalities "that periodically take over and gain control" (Spanos et al., 1984).

The next chapter discusses wider, cultural influences on role enactment as a multiple personality.

CHAPTER 8

Multiple Personality as a Cultural Phenomenon

In the previous chapter it was argued that multiple personality could usefully be understood under the rubric of social role theory. The research of Spanos, in particular, has exposed some of the demand characteristics of situations that might more properly be seen as generating rather than "uncovering" multiple personalities. Here I want to widen the focus from small group influences on behaviour and experience to the role of culture. I will also ask whether a socio-cultural perspective might not be complemented by recourse to more conventional psychiatric classification. Reconciliation between the medical model and more social approaches is nothing new although "cross-cultural" psychiatry seems to occupy an undervalued place in contemporary texts and training courses.

Cross-cultural psychiatry comes in "strong" and "weak" versions which represent the two poles of an absolutist-relativist continuum. The "strong" version posits that psychological disturbances are social creatures, products of the specific culture in which a patient resides. Thus we might hypothesise that different cultures will generate idiosyncratic syndromes. More extremely, we might hypothesise that in some cultures there will be a virtual absence of so-called "mental illness". The "weak" version would have it that all mental disorder has common formal mechanisms and dynamics. One role of culture would be no more than to shape the content and manifestation of universal psychopathologies. Thus, for example, paranoid schizophrenic delusions in technological cultures may involve beliefs about the toxic effects of "rays" from television screens. The delusions of a paranoid schizophrenic in a primitive, tribal culture may take the form of believing that one is under the evil hex of the local witch doctor. Guilt is a common component of depression in some cultures but not in others.

In a sense, the "strong" version sees the role of culture as relatively trivial in much the same way that one could argue that the particular language one speaks is a trivial accident of birth. Pursuing this analogy, what is fundamental is that all languages derive from a finite set of "linguistic universals". The existence of such universal cognitive rules is convincing evidence of the biological underpinnings of the sub-systems of language acquisition. Language is thus construed as species-specific rather than culture-specific. (This does not infer that language is specific to only one species, however.)

The cross-cultural approach to psychopathology looks not only at the behaviour and experience of patients but also at the perception and interpretation of such behaviour and experience by other members of the same culture, notably the professional carers. To what extent, for example, do diagnostic and treatment practices differ between cultures? Relatedly, to what extent does the cultural background of patient, diagnostician and/or therapist influence behaviour in clinical settings?

Illustratively, two studies (Cooper et al., 1972; Kendall, 1975) of the diagnostic practice of British, American and Canadian psychiatrists found striking cross-cultural differences in the incidence of the diagnosis of schizophrenia, ranging from 25% in Britain to 69% in the United States. Differences in the theoretical orientation of training courses, in the usage of technical vocabulary and in taxonomy are some of the (scientifically trivial) factors.

Cultural differences in incidence are also reported. Although depression has been described as the common cold of mental illness, Marsella (1980) has concluded that depression, as defined in Western culture, has a much lower incidence in non-Western societies. African, South American and Asian tribal groups have a higher incidence of hysterical conversion neurosis, but a lower incidence of obsessive-compulsive neurosis, than the population of the United States (Draguns, 1980).

It is essential to point out that a cultural perspective also means curiosity about the influence of such factors as sex differences and social class. In Western cultures, for example, women patients are far more likely to be diagnosed as "hysteric" whereas male patients are more likely to receive the label "psychopath" (e.g. Lerner, 1974).

The absolutist, medical model can easily be reconciled with more sociological approaches provided that one sees cultural factors as doing no more than "fleshing out" organically based syndromes or as furnishing different stage directions for the enactment of what are, essentially, the same roles. Where the two approaches come into conflict is when one posits that, for example, mental disorders are nothing more than cultural artifacts. Such a position is more than mere polemic. It has profound implications for how we deal with psychological distress. To express the issue in crude metaphor, should patients be left in the waiting room while we get on with making Society a healthier place in which to live?

A simple compromise between the culturally relative and species-absolutist approaches to psychological disorder is to accept that some disorders may be universal whilst others are endemic to particular cultures. To insist that all mental illness is no more than a cultural product connives at current evidence on the genetics of schizophrenia or the effectiveness of lithium therapy in alleviating manic–depressive psychosis.

However, syndromes do exist which are manifestly culture-bound. Merskey (1979), for example, refers to Latah (Yap, 1951; 1952), Ainu (Uchimara, cited in Kretschmer, 1948), Amok (Westermeyer, 1972), Pibloktoq (Brill, 1913; Ackernecht, 1948), Wihtigo (Yap, 1951), Voodoo (Sargant, 1957) and Phii Pob (Suwanlert, 1976):

> Malayan women subject to Latah behave compliantly often with echopraxia, echolalia and even coprolalia usually following a sudden fright, such as seeing or stepping on a snake. Imu (Winiariz and Wielawski, 1936) is a virtually identical syndrome seen amongst the Ainu of Japan. Individuals behave wildly and run away in panic normally after seeing snakes, snails or caterpillars. They show echoing and automatic obedience, with occasional loss of consciousness but, unlike the Malay variety, there is no amnesia for the episodes. Amok, which is also found in Malayans, is more typically male and begins after a period when the individual has been withdrawn and brooding. They then suddenly go berserk and will kill several animals or people before either committing suicide or being killed by their fellows. Pibloktoq is a rare form of hysteria found among Eskimos where the (normally) female victim screams and tears at her clothing, shouts obscenities and even eats faeces. She may imitate animal or bird cries and leave the shelter of home to expose herself to the dangers of the ice pack and snowdrifts. Whitigo, a psychiatric illness of the Cree, Ojibway and Salteaux Indians [leads victims to believe that they have] been transformed into a man-eating, giant monster. (Merskey, 1979).

The Voodoo cult of Haiti involves belief in a number of gods who periodically "take possession" of individuals, normally whilst dancing to rhythmic drumming. Phii Pob affects Thailanders who believe that all-powerful spirits, having originated within individuals, then depart from their "hosts" and go on to "possess" others. Patients evidence anxiety and depression as well as motor disturbances such as convulsions and trembling. They also are commonly victim to hallucinations and delusions.

The characteristic "possession" is of three kinds: single instances with no recurrence (akin to "situational crises"), periodic in the setting of an hysterical personality ("possession neuroses"), and cases where acute psychotic symptoms are manifest and the prognosis is good (Suwanlert, 1976).

Langness (1965, 1967) has recorded a syndrome called Negi Negi (which means "deaf") among the Bena bena peoples of New Guinea. Only males between the ages 22 to 32 are affected and the episodes seldom last longer than 24 hours. Victims invariably become temporarily deaf and behave aggressively to their clansmen making threatening gestures, waving clubs and shooting arrows. There is normally amnesia for these acts which appear to be associated with the recent death of a close relative. Another form of behaviour which is almost exclusive to female members of the Bena Bena is "Genefafaili". It normally affects women in mourning who begin to shake violently whereupon they are moved from the house where the body is lying and soot from the fires is put in their hair. The Bena Bena believe that ghosts are responsible for both Negi Negi and Genefafaili but only in the latter do they believe that ghosts possess the victim.

How then, might one appropriately classify such presentations? Their transient and flamboyant nature suggests a diagnosis of hysterical neurosis. However, the degree to which individuals are incapacitated, the delusional and sometimes hallucinatory content of their disorder, and the extremeness of their behavioural deviance, inevitably raises the question of a psychosis. As a way out of this diagnostic impasse what should be more natural than recourse to a label of "hysterical psychosis"? Such nomenclature, however, needs justication and elucidation.

"Hysterical psychosis" is a term which has been usefully revived by Hollender and Hirsch (1964) and further clarified by Hirsch and Hollender (1969). Understandably, the term has had its critics (e.g. Reichard, 1956) because we are used to thinking of hysteria as not only non-psychotic but even as "the mildest form of neurosis" (Richman and White, 1970). Intuitively, however, many clinicians must occasionally have questioned the appropriateness of subsuming the presentations of some of their hysterical patients under the head of "neuroses". The chronically disabling quality of conversion symptoms, the dramatic presentation of those who complain of depersonalisation, the presence of delusions and hallucinations and lack of insight, all can make one wonder about conventional distinctions between neurosis and psychosis.

Matters are not helped by the polymorphous nature of the concept of "hysteria" let alone by a lack of agreement about whether "psychoses" represent extreme degrees of functional disablement or the assumed presence of biological processes.

Apart from Slater's (1965) famous address, when he called the diagnosis of hysteria a "delusion and a snare" which invited psychiatrists to misdiagnose organic and psychotic conditions, both lay and professional usage of the term reveal a bewildering variety of conceptions. For example, Chodoff and Lyons (1958) note that "hysteria" is used in at least the following five ways:

1. A pattern of behaviour habitually exhibited by certain individuals who are said to be hysterical personalities or hysterical characters.
2. A particular kind of psychosomatic symptomatology called conversion hysteria or conversion reaction.
3. A psychoneurotic disorder characterised by phobias and/or certain anxiety manifestations – called anxiety hysteria.
4. A particular psychopathological pattern.
5. A term of opprobrium.

Hollender and Hirsch (1964) saw "hysterical psychosis" as an extreme presentation of hysterical personality disorder with the following characteristics:

1. Sudden and dramatic onset.
2. Precipitation by a profoundly upsetting event or situation.
3. Hallucinations.
4. Delusions.
5. Depersonalisation or bizzare behaviour.
6. Absence of thought disorder or presence of a thought disorder that is circumscribed and transient.

7. Affect tending toward volatility rather than flatness.
8. Acute episode lasting 1–3 weeks,with minimal or no residue at the end of the episode.
9. Greater frequency among individuals regarded as having hysterical characters or hysterical personalities.

Gift, Strauss and Young (1985) studied a sample of 217 first-admission patients with a diagnosis of hysteria and found none who fulfilled all of these criteria. They concluded that the clinical utility of the concept was questionable. However, the most important disqualifying characteristic "was the duration of the episode. For almost all patients, a protracted onset, plus the continuation of significant symptoms after admission, resulted in an episode running much beyond 3 weeks" (Gift et al., 1985).

Steingard and Frankel (1985), however, do find "hysterical psychosis" a clinically useful term. They present the case of a cyclothymic, 17-year-old girl with recurrent visual and auditory hallucinations and a history of disturbed behaviour and a suicide attempt. Their diagnosis was hysterical psychosis consequent upon her father's depressive illness. The authors suggest that one important mechanism for transient or recurrent events of psychotic proportions is the mechanism of dissociation. Their patient proved to be highly hypnotisable and therapy comprised learning control about entering and emerging from her dissociated states. This is clearly reminiscent of Frankel's (1976) notion of the deliberate use of trance as a coping mechanism.

Following the distribution of the film, *The Exorcist*, Bozzuto (1975) reported on the cases of four individuals with no previous psychiatric history. Within a day of seeing the film all four developed paranoid ideas together with delusions about being possessed by the Devil. In the following year I too saw in my outpatient clinic two women, with no psychiatric history, who had been deeply disturbed by the film. They, too, presented with delusions about possession but also complained of delusional perceptions. One said that she was being followed by stray dogs who "made signs which told me that they were agents of Satan." The other reported seeing the Devil's horns sprouting from the heads of horses grazing in a field at the back of her house. Both responded well to brief psychotherapy as was the case with Bozzuto's patients. Although Bozutto terms these episodes "cinematic neuroses", the schizophreniform presentation suggests that they might more appropriately be seen as hysterical psychoses.

From the perspective of family therapy, Richman and White (1970) also find clinical value in the concept although they observe that "the diagnosis of 'hysterical psychosis' has been applied, often apologetically, to patients whose symptoms did not fit the usual nosological categories." Their own usage of the term has been guided by the presence of such factors as:

1. Acute onset and rapid recovery.
2. Absence of schizophrenic thought disorder.
3. A childlike quality in patients combined with a naive flirtatiousness.

4. Impression as "an actor who can take on a part, rather than as someone who becomes the part he is playing."
5. "The central importance of situational and family factors and the role of significant others".

Richman and White immediately go on to cite Langness' (1967) emphasis on the role of cultural factors in hysterical psychosis in primitive societies, "where precipitating incidents, symptomatology, and societal responses all seem to be consistent, predictable and culturally specific."

In the present context, Richman and White's concluding remarks are highly relevant: "We found that each family can be considered hysterogenic in a family-specific way, that psychosis, like conversion, can be an alternative when repression fails, and ... can best be understood in a family context ... [we agree with] Hollender and Hirsch, who emphasise both the specific stress and the personality predisposition [and] the severity of the conflict in these patients, their extreme resort to denial, and the ineffectiveness of their neurotic behaviour in manipulating the environment. Similarly, the severity of the conflicts in our hysterical psychotic families stood out, as compared to those in the families of neurotic patients." These authors go on to note factors common to all their cases: "illness was associated with anxiety related to death, aggression and actual object loss. Every patient was or had been suicidal. In every instance we could determine that the psychotic symptoms were family syntonic. This attitude might be compared to those in societies with socially sanctioned forms of psychotic release, such as running amok."

Hollender and Hirsch recall that Freud's (1894) early formulation of hysteria extended to include psychotic behaviour which he saw as a defence against unbearable ideas and their associated anxieties and guilt. Psychosis was conceptualised as a wish-fulfilling flight from intolerable experience. In a second paper on the psychoneuroses (1896) Freud attributed psychosis to a failure in repression so that current stressors allowed primitive material to erupt as well as modifying ego-regulation of reality. Along with Brody (1961) they suggest that this formulation might well fit an hysterical psychosis.

Descriptively, hysterical psychoses mostly affect women and have an acute and dramatic onset, normally following explicit trauma. Their duration is rarely longer than a matter of weeks although future episodes are not uncommon. They also occur in individuals with hysterical personalities.

In a personal communication, Brody has stated that the term hysterical psychosis seemed occasionally appropriate when the psychological condition, while fulfilling the criteria for a failure in reality testing appeared to have a clear problem-solving or wish-fulfilling function (Hollender and Hirsch, 1964). Brody elaborated that "the tendency to think of 'hysterical psychosis' rather than schizophrenia would be greater when the secondary, interpersonal or adaptive gain from the psychotic behaviour is most obvious." In another personal communication, Alexander has opined that "the term 'hysterical psychosis' is really a telegram-style reference to hysterical states which from the point of view of descriptive symptomatology strongly resemble psychotic states." Similarly, Bond has personally communicated that he has always regarded the differences between schizophrenia and hysterical psychosis as the contact of the patient with the environment, the easily understandable dynamics and the shortness of duration.

Hollender and Hirsch also state that what they term hysterical psychosis often refers to "transient psychosis" (excluding toxic states and acute delirium) described by Bower (1961) as follows: "in transient psychosis the conflict is severe, usually environmental, escape routes are barred, and there usually exists an inability to manipulate or influence the factors contributing to the conflict situation. Neurotic mechanisms are inapplicable and non-goal-directed, and regressive behaviour results."

Amongst the illustrative case studies which Hollender and Hirsch present is a 26-year-old married woman, in the throes of a divorce, who was abandoned by her parents when she gave birth to an illegitimate child. She began to read the Bible fervently, and became progressively more hyperactive and disorganised. Following chlorpromazine therapy she was discharged within a fortnight and 4 months later entered into a turbulent marriage with the father of her child.

Some time later, following a violent argument she was found in a partly filled bath with eyes closed. She said she had drowned but God had revived her and she was now a form of God with a mission to care for women. Once again she recovered rapidly and we are to assume there were no further psychotic episodes.

Hollender and Hirsch suggest that such hysterical psychoses are the end-points of a continuum beginning with hysterical personality. Individuals at risk are those who have developed "antennae" to deal with social situations and who are especially sensitive to social cues. Their life style is characterised by volatility, frequent mood changes and role playing. It is also suggested that early experiences foster "an outlook oriented to 'affective truth' (i.e. it feels or seems right so it is right) instead of to facts, logic and validation." Langness (1967) has noted that primitive peoples, where hysterical psychosis is more commonly reported, are typically non-scientific in orientation, believe in magic and rely on conventional precepts as guides to action. He speculates that their sensitivity to cues derives from the small-scale, intimate, and face-to-face contact which typifies their tribal lives.

In their later paper, Hirsch and Hollender (1969) refined their earlier ideas about hysterical psychosis being the end product of a single process. They propose that hysterical psychoses can be subsumed under three heads; culturally sanctioned behaviour, the appropriation of psychotic behaviour and true psychosis.

Culturally sanctioned behaviour refers to behaviour, which although violent and disturbing, is accepted as an institutionalised means of tension reduction. Freed and Freed (1966), for example, quote a north Indian villager who said of a clanswoman that she "formerly was possessed of a ghost ...but now she is mad." Hirsch and Hollender make the point that we still await a conceptual framework for the transcultural comparative analysis of culture-bound disorders, a field which is ripe for interdisciplinary study.

Under their second head, the appropriation of psychotic behaviour, it is argued that hysterical conversion need not apply uniquely to physical symptoms such as paralyses and anaesthesias. Individuals may also act out a pantomime of psychosis when they cannot express their true feelings and wish to provoke particular responses from others. These enactments derive from their personal understanding, based on hearsay experience, films and books, of psychotic manifestations. These authors see such presentations as distinct from genuine psychotic phenomena because patients "far from being out of contact with reality, are intent on establishing contact, however circuitous the means they adopt to accomplish this. It is important to them that others be aware that they are in the throes of a unique and strange psychological experience, particularly certain significant others ...."

True psychosis is present when there is disruption and breakdown of ego-boundaries and is reminiscent of Freud's (1896) second article on the psychoneuroses. It appears when primitive and largely unconscious materials erupts into awareness with a consequent modification of reality testing. Hirsch and Hollender make the interesting proposition that the cognitive style of the hysteric predisposes them to psychotic breakdown; "a psychological organisation characterised by impressionistic, relatively immediate, and global cognition and by a too quick and insufficient organisation, refinement, and integration of mental contents ... is particularly vulnerable to ego disruption."

Siomopoulos (1971) discusses certain aspects of the psychopathology of the delusional-hallucinatory experiences of hysterical psychosis which seem to distinguish it from schizophrenia.

Angyal (1965) and Fenichel (1945) both thought that hysterical delusions coexisted with good reality contact, and reality-testing was not totally suspended. Patients do not "believe in the ideas and call them 'crazy' " (Fenichel, 1945). Fenichel, however, referred to such patients as borderline hysterics rather than making any connection with hysterical psychosis.

Siomopoulos suggests that hysterical psychotic patients describe their hallucinations somewhat vaguely, reminiscent of the descriptive vagueness of hysterical pains. This is consistent with Szasz (1961) who argued that hysteria is a mode of communication in a non-discursive, pictorial body language. Siomopoulos goes on to contend that "when these patients talk about their 'voices' or 'visions' they communicate thought contents rather than specific perceptual occurrences accessible to recall. In contrast to schizophrenic hallucinations, which represent perceptualisation of thought contents, the hallucinations of hysterical psychosis are thought contents which are communicated as pereptual experiences without having been previously perceptualised." Interestingly, Siomopoulos begins by talking about hysteria in terms of somatic conversions but gradually comes to much the same position as Hirsch and Hollender whereby conversion also includes the appropriation of psychotic behaviour and experience. In other words, the conventional distinction between conversion and dissociative hysterias is deliberately blurred.

In his discussion, Shapiro (1965) and Kuiper (1967) are cited as but two of the clinicians who have observed that hysterics frequently impress as not really believing in their own dramatic presentations. This ability to conjure up the most vivid fantasy worlds, and to act out complex roles therein, whilst at the same time recognising their artificiality is reminiscent of the make-believe worlds of normal children. For Siomopoulos, hysterical psychosis represents a regression to this childlike form of cognitive activity. He suggests that "the delusional ideas of hysterical psychosis constitute a microscopic picture in the area of thought processes of the massive splitting of consciousness that is identified, usually as a variant of conversion hysteria, as personality dissociation ... a similar dissociative thought pattern is present in the hallucinations of hysterical psychosis."

Mallett and Gold (1964) have described a cohort of female patients with a history of visual hallucinations, depression, superficial relationships, physical complaints, sexual problems and feelings of "emptiness". All had been diagnosed, at some time, as schizophrenic but were eventually relabelled as hysteric. These authors suggest that an appropiate diagnosis would have been "pseudo-schizophrenic hysterical syndrome". A number of researchers have wondered whether "hysterical psychosis" might not have been even more appropriate.

Amongst these are Spiegel and Fink (1979) and it will be recalled, from Chapter 6, that David Spiegel has proposed that there is an operationally definable group of individuals who are especially susceptible to hypnotic suggestion, the Grade 5 syndrome. In their 1979 paper, Spiegel and Fink endorse the usefulness of the concept of "hysterical psychosis" and suggest that it can be distinguished from true psychosis through the medium of hypnosis. They note that research since 1964 has pointed to low hypnotisability in schizophrenic populations, whereas high hypnotisability has been noted amongst hysterical patients since Charcot (1890). Hypnotisability, therefore, becomes a useful differential diagnostic indicator and "from this point of view such hysterical symptoms as fugue states, amnesia, and hallucinations are understood as spontaneous, undisciplined trance states. Some individuals, in the face of dramatic stress within their family, at their job, or social pressure of other kinds may succumb to a psychotic form of communication which is different from schizophrenia in phenomenology, course and prognosis" (Spiegel and Fink, 1979).

Spiegel and Fink present two illustrative cases. The first, Michael, was the 15-year-old member of a deeply religious family who believed he was possessed by Satan. Ten weeks before admission he had become involved with his first girl-friend and later he attacked her with a knife. A priest, in whom he confided, told him this was the Devil's work. On admission he said he had no delusions or hallucinations other than that he wondered whether he might be possessed by demons." The ward staff considered him a paranoid schizophrenic but a week after admission he was administered the Hypnotic Induction Profile and proved capable of a profound trance state involving age regression so that the past seemed "as though it were the present". The family were counselled to treat him with calm reassurance, to pay him less attention and to move him from the bedroom he shared with his sexually active sister. The authors posit that his psychosis was a meaningful reaction to his family's religiosity against which he subconsciously rebelled. It was his communication that if they wanted religion then they could have it! In the authors' words, "his illness succeeded in getting him out of the over-sexualised family situation in the short term and then getting him out of his sister's room in the long run ... although he was psychotic and delusional, his affect was atypical in that he was capable of forming good rapport in the intervals between his states of possession, and he showed periods of intense and dramatic affect." Michael responded well to family therapy given a change in his sleeping arrangements and the amount of attention devoted to him by family members. After a 1-year follow-up he was doing well without medication or psychotherapy.

Their second case history revolves around a 31-year-old woman whose symptoms, which included a suicide attempt, were provoked by a sexual advance from a man she had met only recently. She reported that she could "see through" people and she could see flames burning inside certain men. She also recounted how, when driving alone, she had hallucinated a woman with whom she discussed her worries. The woman was very different from the patient in voice, appearance and self-confidence. The patient had a history of headaches, together with low back pain, allergies and "hypoglycemia" with no organic basis. Therapy focused on her inability to feel any real independence following her separation from her husband. She was caught in the bind of wanting to take the initiative to please but, at the same time, doubting her own judgement. She proved to be a Grade-5 subject and by learning to control her entry into and her exit from the trance state she learned to control her anxiety about making decisions without resort to hallucinations and suicide gestures as defences.

Spiegel and Fink argue convincingly that her symptoms were nonverbal communications about her fear of men and, indeed, her own sexuality, together with uncertainty about dealing with sexually loaded, interpersonal situations. Thus trance is used both as differential diagnostic indicator and a therapeutic tool. The latter use of hypnotic imaging is clearly reminiscent of Frankel's (1976) paper on trance as a coping mechanism. Spiegel and Fink suggest that this patient's symptoms were her way of communicating nonverbally her fear of men's sexual advances and her inability to cope with them, as well as with her own sexual desires. They conclude that "because these individuals are so compliant, they can easily slip into a pattern of chronic psychological dysfunction if that is the expectation of their therapist and treating environment". They conclude on the optimistic note that the assessment of hypnotisability may pave the way for selecting a subgroup of psychotic patients who will respond to psychotherapy as opposed to antipsychotic medication.

The revival of interest in hysterical psychosis as a scientifically useful diagnostic category is to be welcomed and I now want to explore, what seems to me, a number of striking similarities between this syndrome and the phenomenon of multiple personality.

Hysterical psychosis subsumes a range of disorders where the sufferers portray a number of common characteristics premorbidly, symptomatically and in treatment response. They tend to have hysterical personalities and a dramatic, even flamboyant presentation. Their cognitive style is a preference for affective truth and for global impression formation rather than analytic thinking modes. They are extraordinarily sensitive to social cues, suggestible, highly hypnotisable and their presentations are frequently reminiscent of the behaviour of hypnotised subjects. They are emotionally volatile, frequently communicate suicidal intent and are prone to merge fantasy with reality. However, despite the intrusions of autistic as opposed to reality thinking, and the presence of hallucinatory and delusional phenomenology and the frequent sense of being "possessed", they retain contact with reality-testing in a way which sharply distinguishes them from schizophrenic patients. Commonly they recognise the "as-if" quality of their psychotic experience whilst paradoxically succumbing to the role demands of their disturbance. One can also recognise the meaningful and manipulative character of their symptoms which show acute onset, are reactive to identifiable environmental stressors, typically have strong sexual content, and include considerable secondary gain. The symptoms readily allow interpretation as attempts to communicate to others their feeling of being trapped in intolerable, ego-threatening situations which push to the limit their resources to cope. Their symptoms permit temporary escape from such trauma as well as permitting the disavowal of responsibility for socially deviant behaviour. Although individual episodes may be short lived they tend to recur with amnesia for earlier attacks. In the treatment situation, unlike other psychoses, they can establish good rapport and the prognosis is favourable. Finally, these psychoses are frequently culturally specific and relatedly are more common in women than men.

The concordance of this description of hysterical psychosis (dubbed, *inter alia* "transient psychosis", "pseudo-schizophrenia" and "cinematic neurosis") and multiple personality is inescapable. Multiple personality, with its striking dissociative aspect, is a conspicuously hysterical disorder and Hollender and Hirsch, amongst other important contributions, have made it clear that "conversion" need not be confined to somatic symptomatology. Multiple personality patients present with acute onset following environmental trauma which are commonly sexually loaded and their alter egos are conspicuously strategic inventions to help them cope with unmanageable stressors. They are manifestly hypnotisable and sensitive to social cueing and although their disorder may endure for many years, the emergence of alter egos is episodic and brief, and the prognosis is good. Amnesia and socially irresponsible behaviour is the norm, together with a degree of phenomenonologial disturbance which has psychotic proportions. Hardly surprising are the difficulties of differential diagnosis given the resemblances of multiple personality syndrome with the hallucinations and delusions of the schizophrenic, the volatile affect of the manic-depressive, the social deviance of the sociopathic personality disorder, the affective psychopathology of certain temporal lobe epileptics, the machinations of the malingerer, and, far from least, the iatrogenic creatures of prolonged, psychoanalytically based therapy which also employs hypnotic suggestion.

The remaining, striking, feature of many hysterical psychoses is their cultural specificity. It will be recalled that my initial impetus to write this monograph was the dramatic incidence of multiple personality syndrome in the United States relative to its virtual absence elsewhere in the world. An extensive canvass of psychologists and psychiatrists in Great Britain produced not a single, unequivocal case of multiple personality, nor do any exist in the UK literature. A Czechoslovakian colleague, consultant psychiatrist Dr Zdenek Boleloulcky, wrote to me to say that in the CSSR multiple personality is "unknown to the present day generation of psychiatrists." There is a similar dearth of cases in New Zealand and Australia. Varma et al. (1981), presenting a single case study of a possession state, write that "no case of double or multiple personality so labelled by a psychiatrist, has been reported from India in the professional literature." It would be absurd to claim that this represents some world-wide survey of the incidence of multiple personality syndrome. It is, however, at least suggestive that we are dealing with a psychological disturbance which is endemic to the United States of America.

At this stage one can only speculate about what features of United States culture might be conducive to multiple personalities. Varma et al. (1981) suggest that "twentieth-century Western man, especially in North America, has shown a special fascination with role playing. The role is adopted with some gain or favourable outcome in mind. The fulfillment of the role may make him act even in a manner contrary to his usual self ... The role adopted, like in a multiple personality ... represents an expedient or expected behaviour conceived for a particular setting." These authors then go on to make the interesting proposition that although multiple personality is a rare condition all over the world, "its even greater rarity in India may be due to the wider acceptance of hysterical possession states and the large variety of potential 'possessors' (deities and spirits)." This emphasis on the high social approval accorded to role playing in the United States does not seem exaggerated. For good or ill, North America is inextricably associated with show business (the business of show) and the film industry in particular. There is a merging of the worlds of entertainment and politics, for example, which is foreign to the European experience. Film stars become politicians and politicians campaign like film stars. When a nation's leaders adopt a particular form of impression management there is likely to be a certain impact on the culture. By comparison, the British member of parliament can seem somewhat staid.

The United States not only loves its movie stars, it also loves its psychiatrists, psychoanalysts and psychologists. The influence and prestige of these professions is far greater than, for example, in Britain. Only part of the explanation lies in their greater numbers (there are less than 2000 clinical psychologists in the UK). The tendency in Britain is still to regard psychology et al. as techniques for dealing with certain forms of mental illness. Ideally, one has recourse to them rarely, if ever, and hopes that the course of therapy will be as brief as possible. It certainly is not something to be noised abroad. Seeing one's psychiatrist is a confidential business rather than dinner party conversation. North Americans seem to have long destigmatised psychotherapy. They have integrated psychology into their daily lives as part of personal growth as well as crisis intervention or treating mental illness. The cost of such psychological sophistication might be an undue tendency to self-analysis and introspection, an undue tendency to act out neurotic roles in order to communicate a heightened sense of bewilderment.

The biographies of Eve and Sybil, and the derivative films have received considerable publicity in the United States and the films are frequently rerun on television. The magazine, *Speaking for Ourselves*, was referred to in the opening chapter. I suggest that, consequentially, there is far more awareness of multiple personality in the United States than in Britain and more source data to provide role models.

Far from least in this cultural scenario are the clinician/investigators themselves. The foregoing monograph has looked at a vast array of evidence for the discrete existence of multiple personality syndrome ranging from laboratory investigations through clinical testimony to self-report. The condition is variously described as of epidemic proportions, as extremely rare and as a chimera. My own strong impression is that the diagnosis of multiple personality owes as much to cultural influence as does its ontogeny. Even accepting its validity as a clinical entity, as a culture-specific, atypical hysterical psychosis presenting in individuals with Grade-5 syndrome premorbid personalities, the highly equivocal evidence suggests that it is grossly overdiagnosed. One should only diagnose multiple personality when there is corroborative evidence that complex and integrated alter egos, with amnesic barriers, existed prior to therapy and emerge without hypnotic intervention by clinicians.

References

Abse, W. (1982). Multiple personality. In A. Roy (Ed.), *Hysteria*. New York: Wiley.

Ackerknecht, E.H. (1948). Medicine and disease among Eskimos. *Ciba Symposia, 10*, 916-921.

Allison, R.B. (1974). A guide to parents: How to raise your daughters to have multiple personalities. *Family Therapy, 1*, 83-88.

Allison, R.B. (1978). On discovering multiplicity. *Sven Tidskr Hypnos, 2*, 4-8.

Allison, R.B. (1984). Difficulties diagnosing the multiple personality syndrome in a death penalty case. *International Journal of Clinical and Experimental Hypnosis, 32*, 102-117.

Allison, R.B. & Schwartz, T. (1980). *Minds in many pieces*. New York: Rawson, Wade.

Allport, G.W. (1955). *Becoming: Basic considerations for a psychology of personality*. New Haven and London: Yale University Press.

Allport, G.W. (1961). *Pattern and growth in personality*. New York: Holt, Rinehart and Winston.

American Psychiatric Association. (1963). *Diagnostic and statistical manual of mental disorders*. (2nd ed.) Washington D.C.: Author.

American Psychiatric Association. (1980). *Diagnostic and statistical manual of mental disorders*. (3rd ed.) Washington D.C.: Author.

Angya, A. (1965). *Neurosis and treatment: A holistic theory*. New York: Wiley.

Aplin, D.Y. & Kane, J.M. (1985). Variables affecting pure tone and speech audiometry in experimentally simulated hearing loss. *British Journal of Audiology, 19*, 219-228.

Azam, E.E. (1887). *Hypnotisme, double conscience et alteration de la personnalite*. Preface de J.M. Charcot, Paris, J.B. Bailliere.

Bahnson, C.B. & Smith, K. (1975). Autonomic changes in a multiple personality. *Psychosomatic Medicine, 37*, 85-86.

Balint, M. (1968). *The basic fault: Therapeutic aspects of regression*. London: Tavistock.

Bannister, D. (1968). The myth of physiological psychology. *Bulletin of the British Psychological Society, 21*, 229-231.

Barbara, D. (1974). Review of 'Sybil', F.S. Schreiber, 1973, Regnery. *American Journal of Psychiatry, 131*, 942-943.

Barbara, D. (1975). Reply to 'Sybil: Grande hysterie or folie a deux?' *American Journal of Psychiatry, 132*, 202-203.

Bear, D. (1979). Temporal lobe epilepsy: A syndrome of sensory-limbic hyperconnection. *Cortex, 15*, 357-384.

Bear, D., Levin, K., North, E. (1980). Case report: Temporal lobe epilepsy. *Journal of Clinical Psychiatry, 41*, 89-95.

Bentov, I. (1977). *Stalking the wild pendulum: On the mechanics of consciousness.* New York: E.P. Dutton Inc.

Berglas, S. & Jones, E.E. (1978). Drug choice as a self-handicapping strategy in response to noncontingent success. *Journal of personality and Social Psychology, 32*, 915-921.

Berman, E. (1977). Multiple personality: Theoretical approaches. *Journal of the Bronx State Hospital, 2*, 99-107.

Berman, E. (1981). Multiple personality: Psychoanalytic perspectives. *International Journal of Psychoanalysis, 62*, 288-300.

Binet, A. (1896). *Alterations of personality.* New York: Appleton.

Bircher-Benner, M. (1933). Der Menschenseele Not, Erkrangung und Gesundung. Zurich: Wendepunkt-Verlag, 2, 288-310.

Bliss, E.L. (1980). Multiple personalities: A report of 14 cases with implications for schizophrenia and hysteria. *Archives of General Psychiatry, 37*, 1388-1397.

Bliss, E.L. (1984a). A symptom profile of patients with multiple personalities, including MMPI results. *Journal of Nervous and Mental Disease, 172*, 197-202.

Bliss, E.L. (1984b). Spontaneous self-hypnosis in multiple personality disorder. *Psychiatric Clinics of North America, 7*, 135-146.

Bliss, E.L. (1986). *Multiple personality, allied disorders and hypnosis.* Oxford: Oxford University Press.

Bliss, E.L. & Jeppsen, E.A. (1985). Prevalence of multiple personality among inpatients and outpatients. *American Journal of Psychiatry, 142*, 250-251.

Bliss, E.L., Larson, E.M. & Nakashima, S.R. (1983). Auditory hallucinations and schizophrenia. *Journal of Nervous and Mental Disease, 171*, 30-33.

Boor, M. (1981). *A case history and comparative study of a multiple personality.* Resources in Education, Counseling, and Personnel Services, Educational Resources Information Center (ERIC) Document Reproduction Service, ED201934, School of Education, University of Michigan, Ann Arbor.

Boor, M. (1982). The multiple personality epidemic: Additional cases and inferences regarding diagnosis, etiology, dynamics and treatment. *Journal of Nervous and Mental Disease, 170*, 302-304.

Boor, M. & Coons, P.M. (1983). A comprehensive bibliography of literature pertaining to multiple personality. *Psychological Reports, 53*, 295-310.

Bower, H.M. (1961). Transient psychosis. In *Proceedings of the Third World Congress of Psychiatry, 2.* Montreal: University of Toronto Press and McGill University Press.

Bozzuto, J.C. (1975). Cinematic neurosis following 'The Exorcist': Report of four cases. *Journal of Nervous and Mental Disease, 161*, 43-48.

Braginsky, B. & Braginsky, D. (1967). Schizophrenic patients in the psychiatric interview: An experimental study of their effectiveness at manipulation. *Journal of Consulting and Clinical Psychology, 31,* 546-551.

Brandsma, J.M. & Ludwig, A.M. (1974). A case of multiple personality: Diagnosis and therapy. *International Journal of Clinical and Experimental Hypnosis, 22,* 216-233.

Braun, B.G. (1983). Psychophysiologic phenomena in multiple personality and hypnosis. *American Journal of Clinical Hypnosis, 26,* 124-137.

Braun, B.G. (1984a). Hypnosis creates multiple personality: Myth or reality? *International Journal of Clinical and Experimental Hypnosis, 32,* 191-197.

Braun, B.G. (1984b). Towards a theory of multiple personality and other dissociative phenomena. *Psychiatric Clinics of North America, 7,* 171-194.

Braun, B.G. & Braun, R.E. (1979). *Clinical aspects of multiple personality.* Paper presented at the meeting of the American Society of Clinical Hypnosis, San Francisco.

Brende, J.O. (1984). The psychophysiologic manifestations of dissociation: Electrodermal responses in a multiple personality patient. *Psychiatric Clinics of North America, 7,* 41-49.

Brende, J.O. & Rinsley, D. (1981). A case of multiple personality with psychological automatisms. *Journal of the American Academy of Psychoanalysis, 9,* 129-151.

Brill, A.A. (1913). Piblokto or hysteria among Peary's Eskimos. *Journal of Nervous and Mental Disease, 40,* 514.

Breuer, J. & Freud, S. (1955). *Studies in hysteria.* London: Hogarth. (originally published in 1895).

Brody, E.B. (1961). *Journal of Nervous and Mental Disease, 133.*

Cameron, N. (1944). *The functional psychoses in personality and the behaviour disorders.* (Ed. J. McV. Hunt), New York: Ronald Press.

Charcot, J.M.(1890). *Oeuvres completes de JM Charcot.* Tome 9, Paris: Lecrosnier et Babe.

Cheek, D.B. & LeCron, L.M. (1968). *Clinical hypnotherapy.* New York: Grune and Stratton.

Chodoff, P. & Lyons, H. (1958). Hysteria, the hysterical personaity and 'hysterical' conversion. *American Journal of Psychiatry, 114,* 734-740.

Clary, W.F., Burstin, K.J, & Carpenter, J.S. (1984). Multiple personality and borderline personality disorder. *Psychiatric Clinics of North America, 7,* 89-100.

Condon, W., Ogston, W.D. & Pacoe, L.V. (1969). Three faces of Eve revisited: A study of transient microstrabismus. *Journal of Abnormal Psychology, 74,* 618-620.

Confer, W.N. & Ables, B.S. (1983). *Multiple Personality: Etiology, diagnosis and treatment.* Human Science.

Congdon, M.H., Hain, J. & Stevenson, I. (1961). A case of multiple personality illustrating the transition from role-playing. *Journal of Nervous and Mental Disease, 132,* 497-504.

Coons, P.M. (1980). Multiple personality: Diagnostic considerations. *Journal of Clinical Psychiatry, 41,* 330-336.

Coons, P.M. (1984). The differential diagnosis of multiple personality. *Psychiatric Clinics of North America, 7,* 51-67.

Coons, P.M. (1986). Treatment progress in 20 patients with multiple personality disorder. *The Journal of Nervous and Mental Disease, 174,* 715-721.

Coons, P.M., Milstein, V. & Marley, C. (1982). EEG studies of two multiple personalities and a control. *Archives of General Psychiatry, 39,* 823-825.

Cooper, J. (1985). Review of 'Anna O. Fourteen contemporary reinterpretations'. Rosenbaum, M. and Muroff, M. (Eds.), 1984, New York: Free press. In *Bulletin of British Psychological Society, 38.*

Cooper, J. (1985). Anna O. *Bulletin of the British Psychological Society, 38,* 155-156.

Cooper, J.E., Kendall, R.E., Gurland, B.J., Sharpe, L., Copeland, J.R.M. & Simon, R.J. (1972). *Psychiatric diagnosis in New York and London: A comparative study of mental hospital admissions*. Maudsley Monograph 20, Oxford University Press.

Cory, C.E. (1919-1920). A divided self. *Journal of Abnormal Psychology, 14*, 281-291.

Cutler, B. & Reed J. (1975). Multiple personality: A single case study with a 15 year follow-up. *Psychological Medicine, 5*, 18-26.

Damgaard, J., Van Benschoten, S. & Fagen, J. (1985). An updated bibliography of literature pertaining to multiple personality. *Psychological Reports, 57*, 131-137.

Danesino, A., Daniels, J. & McLaughlin, T.J. (1979). Jo-Jo, Josephine, and Joanne: A study of multiple personality by means of the Rorschach test. *Journal of Personality Assessment, 43*, 300-313.

DeGree, C.E. & Snyder, C.R. (1985). Adler's psychology (of use) today: Personal history of traumatic life events as a self-handicapping strategy. *Journal of Personality and Social Psychology, 48*, 1512-1519.

Dimond, S.J. (1979). Symmetry and asymmetry in the vertebrate brain. In D.A. Oakley and H.C. Plotkin (Eds.) , *Brain, Behaviour and Evolution*, 189-218, London: Methuen.

Dixon, N.F. (1981). *Preconscious processing*. Chichester: Wiley.

Dixon, N.F. & Henley, S.H.A. (1980). Without awareness. In M.A. Jeeves (Ed.), *Psychological Survey 3*, 31-50. London: George Allen and Unwin.

Draguns, J. (1980). Psychological disorders of clinical severity. In H. Triondis & J. Draguns (Eds.), *Handbook of cross cultural psychology: Psychopathology*. Boston: Allyn and Bacon.

Ellenberger, H.F. (1970). *The discovery of the unconscious: The history and evolution of dynamic psychiatry*. New York: Basic Books.

Ellenberger, H.F. (1972). 'The story of Anna O.', a critical review of new data. *History of the Behavioural Sciences, 8*, 267-279.

Eysenck, H.J. (1960). A rational system of diagnosis and therapy in mental illness. In, *Progress in Clinical Psychology, 4*, 46-64, New York: Grune and Stratton.

Eysenck, H.J. (1958). Anna O. *Bulletin of the British Psychological Society, 38*, 82-83.

Fairbairn, W.R.D. (1952). *An object relations theory of the personality*. New York: Basic Books.

Farber, I. (1975). Sane and insane: Constructions and misconstructions. *Journal of Abnormal Psychology, 84*, 589-620

Fenichel, O. (1945). *The psychoanalytic theory of neurosis*. New York: Norton.

Fisher, R.A. (1958). *Statistical methods for research workers*. New York: Hafner.

Forsyth, D. (1939). The case of a middle-aged embezzler. *British Journal of Medical Psychology, 18*, 141-153.

Frank, J.D. (1973). *Persuasion and healing*. New York: Schoken Books.

Frankel, F.H. (1976). *Hypnosis: Trance as a coping mechanism*. New York: Plenum.

Freud, S. (1955). The ego and the id. (Vol. 19). In J. Strachey (Ed. and Trans.), *The Standard Edition of the Complete Works of Sigmund Freud*. London: Hogarth. (Original publication, 1923).

Freud, S. (1964). Splitting of the ego in the process of defence. (Vol. 23). In J. Strachey (Ed. and Trans.), *The Standard Edition of the Complete works of Sigmund Freud*. London: Hogarth. (Original publication, 1938).

Freud, S. (1948). *The defence neuropsychoses. Collected papers, 1, 59*, London: Hogarth Press. (Original publication, 1894).

Freud, S. (1948). Further remarks on the defence neuropsychoses. *Collected papers, 1, 155*, London: Hogarth Press. (Original publication, 1896).

Gellhorn, E. & Kiely, W.F. (1972). Mystical states of consciousness: Neurophysiological and clinical aspects. *Journal of Nervous and Mental Disease, 154*, 399-405.

Gift, T., Strauss, J. & Young, Y. (1985). Hysterical psychosis: An empirical approach. *American Journal of Psychiatry, 142*, 345-347.

Gill, M.M & Brenman, M. (1959). *Hypnosis and related states: Psychoanalytic studies in regression.* New York: International Universities Press.

Goffman, E. (1969). *The presentation of self in everyday life.* Allen Lane, The Penguin Press.

Gough, H.G. & Heilbrun, A.B. (1965). *The adjective check list manual.* Palo Alto, Calif.: Consulting Psychology Press.

Greaves, G. (1980). Multiple personality; 165 years after Mary Reynolds. *Journal of Nervous and Mental Disease, 168*, 577-596.

Grosz, H.J. & Zimmerman, J. (1965). Experimental analysis of hysterical blindness. *Archives of General Psychiatry, 13*, 255-260.

Gruenewald, D. (1971). Hypnotic techniques without hypnosis in the treatment of dual personality. *Journal of Nervous and Mental Disease, 153*, 41-46.

Gruenewald, D. (1977a). Diagnosis and treatment of multiple personality. *International Journal of Clinical and Experimental Hypnosis, 26*, 1-8.

Gruenewald, D. (1977b). Multiple personality and splitting phenomena: A reconceptualisation. *Journal of Nervous and Mental Diseases, 164*, 385-393.

Gruenewald, D. (1978). Analogues of multiple personality in psychosis. *International Journal of Clinical and Experimental Hypnosis, 26*, 1-8.

Gruenewald, D. (1984). On the nature of multiple personality: Comparisons with hypnosis. *International Journal of Clinical and Experimental Hypnosis, 32*, 170-190.

Harriman, P.L. (1942). The experimental induction of a multiple personality. *Psychiatry, 5*, 179-186.

Harriman, P.L. (1943). A new approach to multiple personality. *American Journal of Orthopsychiatry, 13*, 638-643.

Hartmann, H. (1958). *Ego psychology and the problem of adaptation.* New York: International Universities Press. (Original publication, 1939).

Herzog, A. (1984). On multiple personality: Comments on diagnosis, etiology, and treatment. *International Journal of Clinical and Experimental Hypnosis, 32*, 170-190.

Hilgard, E.R. (1977). *Divided consciousness: Multiple controls in human thought and action.* New York: Wiley.

Hirsch, S.J. & Hollender, M.H. (1969). Hysterical psychosis: Clarification of the concept. *American Journal of Psychiatry, 125*, 909-915.

Hirschmuller, A. (1978). Physiologie und Psychoanalyse im Leben und Werk Joseph Breuers. *Jahrbuch der Psychoanalyse, Supplement 4.* Bonn: Huber.

Hollender, M.H. & Hirsch, S.J. (1964). Hysterical psychosis. *American Journal of Psychiatry, 120*, 1066-1074.

Horevitz, R.P. & Braun B.G. (1984). Are multiple personalities borderline? *Psychiatric Clinics of North America, 7*, 69-88.

Horowitz, M.J. & Becker S.S. (1972). Cognitive reponse to stress: Experimental studies of a compulsion to repeat trauma. In R.R. Hall-Holt and E. Peterfreund (Eds.), *Psychoanalysis and Contemporary Science: An Annual of Integrative and Interdisciplinary Studies.* New York: MacMillan.

Horton, P. & Miller, D. (1972). The etiology of multiple personality. *Comprehensive Psychiatry, 13*, 151-159.

James, W. (1890). *The principles of psychology. 2 vols.* New York: Holt.

Janet, P. (1889). *L'automatisme psychologique.* Paris: Alcan.

Janet, P. (1907). *The major symptoms of hysteria.* New York: MacMillan.

Jeans, R.F. (1976a). The three faces of Evelyn: A case report. I. An independently validated case of multiple personality. *Journal of Abnormal Psychology, 85*, 249-255.

Jeans, R.F. (1976b). The three faces of Evelyn: A case study. Part III. Reactions to the blind analysis. *Journal of Abnormal Psychlogy, 85*, 271-275.

Jersild, A.T., Markey, F.V. & Jersild, C.L. (1933). Children's fears, dreams, wishes. *Child development Monograph, 12.* New York: Columbia University Teachers' College.

Jones, E.E. & Berglas, S. (1978). Control of attributions about the self through self-handicapping strategies: The appeal of alcohol and the role of underachievement. *Personality and Social Psychology Bulletin, 4*, 200-206.

Kahr, B.E. (1985). Anna O. *Bulletin of the British Psychological Society, 38*, May, 156.

Kampman, R. (1976). Hypnotically induced multiple personality: An experimental study. *International Journal of Clinical and Experimental Hypnosis, 24*, 215-227.

Kelly, G.A. (1955). *The psychology of personal constructs. Vols. I and II.*, New York: Norton.

Kendell, R.E. (1975). The role of diagnosis in psychiatry. *Journal of Consulting and Clinical Psychology.* Oxford: Blackwell Scientific Publications.

Kendell, R.E. (1983). Hysteria. In *Handbook of Psychiatry, vol. 4, The Neuroses and Personality Disorders* (Ed. G.F.M. Russell & I.A. Hersov), 232-246. Cambridge: Cambridge University Press.

Kennedy, A. (1946). Compensation neurosis. *Compensation Medicine, 1*, 19-24.

Kernberg, O.F. (1976). *Borderline conditions and pathological narcissism.* New York: Jason Aronson.

Keverne, E.B. (1983). Pheromones. In J. Nicholson and B. Foss (Eds.) , *Psychological Survey, 4*, 247-265, Leicester: The British Psychological Society.

Keyes, D. (1981). *The minds of Billy Milligan.* New York: Random House.

Kirshner, L.A. (1973). Dissociative reaction: An historical review and clinical study. *Acta Psychiatrica Scandinavia, 49*, 698-711.

Kjervik, D. (1979). Dual personality: Assessment and reintegration. *Journal of Psychiatric Nursing, 17*, 28-32.

Kluft, R.P. (1982). Varieties of hypnotic interventions in the treatment of multiple personality. *American Journal of Clinical Hypnosis, 24*, 230-240.

Kluft, R.P. (1984). Treatment of multiple personality disorder: A study of 33 cases. *Psychiatric Clinics of North America, 7*, 9-29.

Kluft, R.P. (1986). High-functioning multiple personality patients: Three cases. *The Journal of Nervous and Mental Disease, 174*, 722-726.

Kohlenberg, R.J. (1973). Behavioristic approach to multiple personality: A case study. *Behavior Therapy, 4*, 137-140.

Kohut, H. (1971). *The analysis of the self.* New York: International Universities Press.

Kreitman, N., Sainsbury, P., Morrissey, J., Towers, J., & Scrivener, J. (1961). The reliability of psychiatric assessment: An analysis. *Journal of Mental Science, 107*, 887-908.

Kretschmer, E. (1961). *Hysteria, reflex and instinct.* Stuttgart, 1948. Trans. Baskin, V. and W., London: Peter Owen.

Kuiper, P. (1967). *On being genuine and other essays.* New York: Basic books.

Lader, M. & Sartorius, N. (1968). Anxiety in patients with hysterical conversion symptoms. *Journal of Neurology Neurosurgery and Psychiatry, 31*, 490-495.

Lacroix, J. & Comper, P. (1979). Lateralization in the electrodermal system as a function of cognitive/hemispheric manipulations. *Psychophysiology, 16*, 116-129.

Langness, L.L. (1965). Hysterical psychosis in the New Guinea highlands: A Bena Bena example. *Psychiatry, 28*, 258-277.

Langness, L.L. (1967). Hysterical psychosis: The cross-cultural evidence. *American Journal of Psychiatry, 124*, 47-56.

Lancaster, E. (1958). *The final face of Eve.* McGraw-Hill, New York.

Larmore, K., Ludwig, A.M. & Cain, R.L. (1977). Multiple personality: An objective case study. *British Journal of Psychiatry, 131*, 35-40.

Lasky, R. (1978). The psychoanalytic treatment of a case of multiple personality. *Psychoanalytic Review, 65*, 353-380.

Leavitt, M.C. (1947). A case of hypnotically produced secondary and tertiary personalities. *Psychoanalytic Review, 34*, 274-295.

LeDoux, J.E., Wilson, D.H. & Gazzaniga, M.S. (1979). Beyond commissurotomy: Clues to consciousness. In M.S. Gazzaniga (Ed.), *Handbook of Behavioural Neurobiology, vol. 2*, 543-554. New York: Plenum Press.

Lerner, H.E. (1974). The hysterical personality: A woman's disease. *Comprehensive Psychiatry, 15*, 157-164.

Lord, E. (1950). Experimentally induced variations in Rorschach performance. *Psychological Monographs, 64*, no. 316.

Ludwig, A.M. (1966). Altered states of consciousness. *Archives of General Psychiatry, 15*, 225-234.

Ludwig, A.M., Brandsma, J.M., Wilbur, C.B., Bendfeldt, F. & Jameson, D.H. (1972). The objective study of a multiple personality, or, are four heads better than one? *Archives of General Psychiatry, 26*, 298-310.

McDougall, W. (1926). *Outline of abnormal psychology.* New York: Scribner.

McGuire, R.J. (1973). Classification and the problem of diagnosis. In H.J. Eysenck (Ed.), *Handbook of Abnormal Psychology.* London: Pitman Medical.

McKellar, P. (1979). *Mindsplit: The psychology of multiple personality disorder and the dissociated self.* London: Dent & Sons.

MacCorquodale, K. & Meehl, P.E. (1948). On a distinction between hypothetical constructs and intervening variables. *Psychological Review, 55*, 95-107.

Mallett, B.L. & Gold, S. (1964). A pseudoschizophrenic hysterical syndrome. *British Journal of Medical Psychology, 37*, 59-70.

Marmer, S.S. (1980). Psychoanalysis of multiple personality. *International Journal of Psychoanalysis, 61*, 439-459.

Marsella, A. (1980). Depressive experience of disorder across cultures. In H. Triandis & J. Droguns (Eds.), *Handbook of Cross Cultural Psychology: Psychopathology.* Boston: Allyn and Bacon.

Martin, A.E. (1909). The occurrence of remissions and recovery in tuberculous meningitis. *Brain, 32*, 209.

Masters, W.H. & Johnson, V.E. (1970). *Human sexual inadequacy.* Boston: Little Brown.

Mathew, R.J., Jack, R.A. & Scott West, W. (1985). Regional cerebral blood flow in a patient with multiple personality. *American Journal of Psychiatry, 142*, 504-506.

Mayer-Gross, W., Slater, E. & Roth, M. (1960). *Clinical Psychiatry.* London: Cassell and Co.

Merskey, H. (1979). *The analysis of hysteria*. London: Bailliere Tindall.

Mesulam, M.M. (1981). Dissociative states with abnormal temporal lobe EEG: Multiple personality and the illusion of possession. *Archives of Neurology, 38,* 176-181.

Meyer, J.S. (1978). Improved method for noninvasive measurement of regional cerebral blood flow by [133]Xenon inhalation, part II: Measurements in health and disease. *Stroke, 9,* 205-210.

Miller, E. (1988). Defining hysterical symptoms. *Psychological Medicine, 18,* 275-277.

Miller, G.A., Galanter, E. & Pribram, K.H. (1960). *Plans and the structure of behaviour*. New York: Holt, Rinehart and Winston.

Moseley, A.L. (1953). Hypnogogic hallucinations in relation to accidents, abstracted. *American Psychologist, 8,* 8.

Morselli, G.E. (1930). Sulla dissazione mentale. *Rivista Sperimentale di Freniatria,* 209-322.

Neisser, U. (1966). *Cognitive psychology*. New York: Appleton-Century- Crofts.

Oakley, D.A. & Eames L.C. (1985). The plurality of consciousness. In D.A. Oakley (Ed.), *Brain and Mind*. London and New York: Methuen.

Orne, M.T. (1959). The nature of hypnosis: Artefact and essence. *Journal of Abnormal and Social Psychology, 58,* 277-299.

Orne, M.T., Dinges, D.F. & Orne E.C. (1984). On the differential diagnosis of multiple personality in the forensic context. *International Journal of Clinical and Experimental Hypnosis, 32,* 118-169.

Osgood, C.E. (1952). The nature and measurement of meaning. *Psychological Bulletin, 49,* 192-237.

Osgood, C.E. & Luria, Z. (1954). A blind analysis of a case of multiple personality using the semantic differential. *Journal of Abnormal and Social Psychology, 49,* 579-591.

Osgood, C.E. & Luria, Z. (1957). Introduction. In C.H. Thigpen and H.M. Cleckley, *The three faces of Eve*. New York: Fawcett.

Osgood, C.E., Luria, Z, & Smith, S.W. (1976). The three faces of Evelyn: A case report. Part II. A blind analysis of another case of multiple personality using the semantic differential technique. *Journal of Abnormal Pschology, 85,* 256-270.

Pilowsky, I. (1969). Abnormal illness behaviour. *British Journal of Medical Psychology, 42,* 347-351.

Pines, M. (1978). Invisible playmates. *Psychology Today, 12, 38.*

Pohl, R. (1977). Multiple personality in a middle-aged woman. *Psychiatric Opinion, 14,* 35-39.

Price, J. & Hess, N. (1979). Behaviour therapy as precipitant and treatment in a case of dual personality. *Australian and New Zealand Journal of Psychiatry, 13,* 63-66.

Prince, M. (1906). *The dissociation of a personality*. New York and London: Longmans, Green & Co.

Putnam, F.W. (1984). The psychophysiologic investigation of multiple personality disorder: A review. *Psychiatric Clinics of North America, 7,* 31-39.

Putnam, F.W., Buchsbaum, M., Howland, F. (1982). Evoked potentials in multiple personality disorder. Paper presented at the annual meeting of the American Psychiatric Association. *New Research Abstract, 137.*

Putnam, F.W., Guroff, J.J., Silberman, E.K., Barban, L. & Post, R.M. (1986). The clinical phenomenology of multiple personality disorder: Review of 100 recent cases. *Journal of Clinical Psychiatry, 47,* 285-293.

Reichard, S. (1956). A reexamination of 'Studies in Hysteria'. *Psychoanalytic Quarterly, 25,*

155-177.

Rendon, M. (1977). The dissociation of dissociation. *International Journal of Social Psychiatry, 23* 240-243.

Richman, J. & White, H. (1970). A family view of hysterical psychosis. *American Journal of Psychiatry, 127,* 280-285.

Rosenbaum, M. (1980). The role of the term schizophrenia in the decline of diagnoses of mutiple personality. *Archives of General Psychiatry, 37,* 1383-1385.

Rosenbaum, M. & Weaver, G.M. (1980). Dissociated states: Status of a case after 38 years. *Journal of Nervous and Mental Disease, 61,* 577-596.

Rosehan, D. (1973). On being sane in insane places. *Science, 180,* 365-369.

Saltman, V. & Solomon, R.S. (1982). Incest and the multiple personality. *Psychological Reports, 50,* 1127-1141.

Sarbin, T.R .& Andersen, M.L (1967). Role-theoretical analysis of hypnotic behaviour. In J.E. Gordon (Ed.), *Handbook of Clinical and Experimental Hypnosis* (pp.319-344). New York: MacMillan.

Sargant, W. (1957). *Battle for the mind.* London: Pan Books.

Schenk, L. & Bear, D. (1981). Multiple personality and related dissociative phenomena in patients with temporal lobe epilepsy. *American Journal of Psychiatry, 138,* 1311-1316.

Schreiber, F.R. (1973). *Sybil.* Chicago: Regnery.

Schultz, R., Braun, B.G. & Kluft, R.P. (1985). *Creativity and the imaginary companion phenomenon: Prevalence and phenomenology in MPD.* Paper presented at the Second International Conference on Multiple Personality/Dissociative States. Chicago, October. 1985

Shapiro, D. (1965). *Neurotic styles.* New York: Basic Books.

Shelley, W.B. (1981). Dermatitis artefacta induced in a patient by one of her multiple personalities. *British Journal of Dermatology, 105,* 587-589.

Silberman, E.K., Weingartner, H., Braun, B.G. & Post, R.M. (1985). Dissociative states in multiple personality disorder: A quantitative study. *Psychiatry Research, 15,* 253-260.

Siomopoulos, V. (1971). Hysterical psychosis: Psychopathological aspects. *British Journal of Medical Psychology, 44,* 95-100.

Sizemore, C.C. & Pittillo, E.S. (1977). *I'm Eve!* Garden City, New York: Doubleday.

Slater, E. (1965). Diagnosis of 'hysteria'. *British Medical Journal, 1,* 1395-1399.

Smith, J., & Sager, E. (1971). Multiple personality. *Journal of Medical Sociology of New Jersey, 68,* 717-719.

Smith, R.D., Buffington, P. & McCard, R. (1982). *Multiple Personality: Theory, diagnosis, and treatment.* New York: Irvington.

Smith, T.W., Snyder, C.R. & Perkins, S.C. (1983). The self-serving function of hypochondriacal complaints: Physical symptoms as self-handicapping strategies. *Journal of Personality and Social Psychology, 44,* 787-797.

Snyder, C.R. & Smith, T.W. (1982). Symptoms as self-handicapping strategies: The virtues of old wine in a new bottle. In G. Weary and H.L. Mirels (Eds.), *Integrations of Clinical and Social Psychology.* Oxford: Oxford University Press.

Solomon, R.S. & Solomon V. (1982). Differential diagnosis of multiple personality. *Psychological Reports, 51,* 1187-1194.

Spanos, N.P., Radtke, H.L., Hodgins, D.C., Stam, H.J. & Bertrand, L.D. (1983). The Carleton University responsiveness to suggestion scale: Normative data and psychometric properties. *Psychological Reports, 53,* 523-535.

Spanos, N.P., Radtke, H.L. & Bertrand, L.D. (1984). Hypnotic amnesia as a strategic enactment: Breaching amnesia in highly susceptible subjects. *Journal of Personality and Social Psychology, 47*, 1155-1169.

Spanos, N.P., Weekes, J.R., & Bertrand, L.D. (1985). Multiple personality: A social psychological perspective. *Journal of Abnormal Psychology, 94*, 362-376.

Spanos, N.P., Weekes, J.R., Menary, E., & Bertrand, L.D. (1986). Hypnotic interview and age regression procedures in the elicitation of multiple personality symptoms: A simulation study. *Psychiatry, 49*, 298-311.

Sperry, R.W., Zaidel, E. & Zaidel, D. (1979). Self-recognition and social awareness in the disconnected minor hemisphere. *Neuropsychologia, 17*, 153-166.

Spiegel, D. (1984). Multiple personality as a post-traumatic stress disorder. *Psychiatric Clinics of North America, 7*, 101-109.

Spiegel, D. & Fink, R. (1979). Hysterical psychosis and hypnotisability. *American Journal of Psychiatry, 136*, 777-781.

Spiegel, H. (1974). The grade 5 syndrome: The highly hypnotisable person. *International Journal of Clinical and Experimental Hypnosis, 22*, 303-319.

Spitzer, R. (1975). A critique of Rosenhan's "On being sane in insane places". *Journal of Abnormal Psychology, 84*, 462-474.

Spitzer, R.L., Endicott, J.E., & Gibbon, M. (1979). Crossing the border into borderline personality and borderline schizophrenia. The development of criteria. *Archives of General Psychiatry, 36*, 17-24.

Steingard, S. & Frankel, F. (1985). Dissociation and psychotic symptoms. *American Journal of Psychiatry, 142*, 953-955.

Stern, C.R. (1984). The etiology of multiple personalities. *Psychiatric Clinics of North America, 7*, 149-159.

Sutcliffe, J.P. & Jones, J. (1962). Personal identity, multiple personality, and hypnosis. *International Journal of Clinical and Experimental Hypnosis, 10*, 231-269.

Suwanlert, S. (1976). Neurotic and psychotic states attributed to Thai 'Phii Pob' spirit possession. *Australian and New Zealand Journal of Psychiatry, 10*, 119-123.

Szasz, T.S. (1961). *The myth of mental illness: Foundations of a theory of personal conduct.* New York: Hoeber-Harper.

Taylor, W.S. & Martin, M.F. (1944). Multiple Personality. *Journal of Abnormal and Clinical Psychology, 39*, 281-300.

Thigpen, C.H., & Cleckley, H.M. (1954). A case of multiple personality. *Journal of Abnormal and Social Psychology, 49*, 135-151.

Thigpen, C.H. & Cleckley, H.M. (1957). *The three faces of Eve.* New York: McGraw-Hill.

Thigpen, C.H. & Cleckley, H.M. (1984). On the incidence of multiple personality disorder. *International Journal of Clinical and Experimental Hypnosis, 32*, 63-66.

Thornton, E.M. (1983). *Freud and cocaine.* London: Blond & Briggs.

Thornton, E.M. (1985). 'Anna O.' (Berthe Pappenheim). *Bulletin of the British Psychological Society, 38*, 264-265.

Tulving, E. (1978). Relation between encoding specificity and levels of processing. In L.S. Cermak and F.M. Craik (Eds.), *Levels of processing and human memory.* Hillsdale, N.J.: Lawrence Erlbaum Associates Inc.

Varma, V.K., Bouri, M. & Wig, N.N. (1981). Multiple personality in India: Comparison with hysterical possession state. *American Journal of Psychotherapy, 35, 1.*

Vernon, P.E. (1964). *Personality assessment: A critical survey.* Methuen.

Victor, G.V. (1975). Sybil: Grande hysterie or folie a deux? *American Journal of Psychiatry, 132*, 202.

Wagner, E.E. (1971). Structural analysis: a theory of personality based on projective techniques. *Journal of Personality Assessment, 35*, 422-435.

Wagner, E.E. (1978). A theoretical explanation of the dissociative reaction and a confirmatory case presentation. *Journal of Personality Assessment, 42*, 312-316.

Wagner, E.E. (1981). *The interpretation of projective test data* pp.185-204. Springfield: Thomas.

Wagner, E.E., & Heise, M. (1974). A comparison of Rorschach records of three multiple personalities. *Journal of Personality Assessment, 38*, 308-331.

Watkins, J.G. (1976). Ego states and the problem of responsibility. A psychological analysis of the Patty Hearst case. *Journal of Psychiatric Law, 4*, 471-489.

Watkins, J.G. (1984). The Bianchi (L.A. Hillside Strangler) case: Sociopath or multiple personality. *International Journal of Clinical and Experimental Hypnosis, 32*, 67-101.

Watkins, J.G. & Stauffacher, J.C. (1952). An index of pathological thinking in the Rorschach. *Journal of Projective Techniques and Personality Assessment, 16*, 276-286.

Watkins, J.G. & Watkins, H. (1980). Ego states and hidden observers. *Journal of Altered States of Consciousness, 5*, 3-18.

Wechsler, D. (1945). A standardised memory scale for clinical use. *Journal of Psychology, 19*, 87-95.

Wechsler, D. (1958). *The measurement and appraisal of adult intelligence.* Baltimore: Williams and Wilkins Co.

Weingartner, H., Adefris, W., Eich. J.E. (1976). Encoding-imagery specifically in alcohol state dependent learning. *Journal of Experimental Psychology, 2*, 83-87.

Weitzenhoffer, A.M., & Hilgard, E.R. (1962). *Stanford Hypnotic Susceptibility Scale, Form C.* Palo Alto, California, Consulting Psychologists Press.

Westermeyer, J.A. (1972). A comparison of amok and other homicide in Laos. *American Journal of Psychiatry, 129*, 703-708.

White, R.W. (1941). A preface to the theory of hypnotism. *Journal of Abnormal and Social Psychology, 36*, 477-505.

Wilbur, C.B. (1984). Multiple personality and child abuse. *Psychiatric Clinics of North America, 7*, 3-7.

Winer, D. (1978). Anger and dissociation: A case study of multiple personality. *Journal of Abnormal Psychology, 87*, 368-372.

Winiariz, W. & Wielawski, J. (1936). Imu-a psychoneurosis occurring among Ainus. *Psychoanalytic Review, 23*, 181-186.

Yap, P.M. (1951). Mental disease peculiar to certain cultures: A survey of comparative psychiatry. *Journal of Mental Science, 97*, 313-327.

Yap, P.M. (1952). The Latah reaction: Its pathodynamics and nosological position. *Journal of Mental Science, 98*, 515-564.

Author Index

Subject Index